14-MINUTE METABOLIC WORKOUTS

The Fastest, Most Effective Way to Lose Weight and Get Fit

JASON R. KARP, PH.D.

T0040263

Skyhorse Publishing

Skyhorse Publishing books may be purchased in bulk at special discounts for sales promotion, corporate gifts, fund-raising, or educational purposes. Special editions can also be created to specifications. For details, contact the Special Sales Department, Skyhorse Publishing, 307 West 36th Street, 11th Floor, New York, NY 10018 or info@skyhorsepublishing.com.

Skyhorse® and Skyhorse Publishing® are registered trademarks of Skyhorse Publishing, Inc.®, a Delaware corporation.

Visit our website at www.skyhorsepublishing.com.

10 9 8 7 6 5 4 3 2 1

Library of Congress Cataloging-in-Publication Data is available on file.

Interior photos by Jamie Dickerson of J.Dixx Photography.

Cover design by Tom Lau
Cover photo credit: iStock

ISBN: 978-1-5107-1794-7
Ebook ISBN: 978-1-5107-1795-4
Printed in the United States of America

ALSO BY JASON KARP

Run Your Fat Off
The Inner Runner
Running a Marathon For Dummies
Running for Women
101 Winning Racing Strategies for Runners
101 Developmental Concepts & Workouts for Cross Country Runners
How to Survive Your PhD

DEDICATION

To my parents,
Muriel and Monroe,
who taught me many lessons, including the value of time.

TABLE OF CONTENTS

ACKNOWLEDGMENTS

This book would not have been written if not for many people, primary among them my agent, Grace Freedson. Thank you for all the opportunities you have brought me. It has been nine years and eight books since I received your letter in my mailbox offering to represent me. I'm grateful you were willing to take a chance.

I'd also like to thank . . .

Jack Karp, my twin brother, for your support. You are the most talented writer I know. You inspire me every day to view writing as art, and to relentlessly work at the craft until I get it right.

Julie Ganz, editor at Skyhorse Publishing. Your skills have helped shape this book into something that can help millions of people get fit and save time.

Tom Lau, the book's cover designer, for creating a bold and appealing cover that makes the book fly off the shelf.

Madeleine Ball, the publicist at Skyhorse, for all your efforts to get the book into the public's hands.

Jamie Dickerson, owner of J.Dixx Photography, for your awesome photos that bring to life what I described in words.

Martha Carbajal Moreno, for serving as the book's model, adding beauty to the pages and precision to the exercises. Without you, this book would be just a collection of random exercise instructions.

Brett and Kera Murphy, owners of La Jolla Sports Club, for hosting the photo shoot. Your gym provided a great venue for classic and creative shots.

All my friends, acquaintances, and followers, both in person and in social media, for understanding the sacrifices one must make to write books.

WARM-UP

Beginning in the seventh grade, I became fascinated with time—specifically how fast it goes and how each year seems to go by faster than the previous year. When I once shared my perception of time with my ninety-year-old grandmother, she said, "Just wait until you're eighty." I'm still far from eighty, so I can only imagine how fast time will go by then. It likely will go by in no time at all. Even now, each second that comes is gone just as fast, leaving us with only future and past. The advice to "stay present in the moment" becomes impossible.

Time is perhaps the main influencer of how much people exercise. People claim they never have enough of it. But as Albert Einstein, the expert of time itself, proved, time is relative. "Time has no independent existence," he said, "apart from the order of events by which we measure it." In other words, everyone has 14 minutes.

As a personal trainer in a gym a number of years ago, I was talking to one of the members as she rode a stationary bike alongside her workout buddies. While I was explaining how she and her friends could get better results from their workouts, I sensed that she wasn't listening. Perhaps she didn't care for the advice of a young, scrawny-looking runner in cotton sweatpants. A few days later, I saw her again when I was about to go for a run. Seeing me for the first time in my running shorts, she enthusiastically asked, "How can I get legs like yours?" Smiling, I joked, "So, you want me for my body rather than for my mind?"

Everyone wants nice legs. Although it took me a lot longer than 14 minutes to get such nice legs, I've spent much of the last thirty years appreciating the impact that short workouts can have and creating workouts that can make you extremely fit in a short time. *14-Minute Metabolic Workouts* is the solution to everyone's time problem, giving you great results in 14 minutes or less. If you're a skeptical person like me, you may be thinking, *Can I really get fit in just 14 minutes?* You bet your biceps and buttocks you can, if you focus and do it right. *14-Minute Metabolic Workouts* shows you how.

This book includes a variety of compact, science-based workouts that you can do at the gym, at home, or outside. These workouts target the five components of physical fitness—cardiovascular endurance, muscular endurance, muscular strength, body composition, and flexibility. Among these pages, you'll find cardio and sprint intervals; muscular strength, power, and endurance workouts; circuits; plyometrics; and flexibility workouts. For the final chapter, I put all the workouts together in a five-course menu to create a training program for you.

Why 14 minutes? Because it's precise. You pay attention. You focus on the effort because you know the time will be gone as fast as it arrived.

Enjoy the time.

CHAPTER 1

CARDIO WORKOUTS

The ancient Greeks may have been the first to acknowledge the existence of the heart, which they named *kardia*. Aristotle identified the heart as the most important organ of the body and believed that it was the center of man's soul. I'm not sure if my soul is linked to my heart or not, but the heart is certainly linked to my life, as it is to yours, since its only responsibility is to deliver blood and oxygen to all of your organs to sustain life. It is always working, from before you're born until you die.

Despite the attention our society gives to the muscles on your legs, arms, and abs, your heart is where life lives. How well your cardiovascular system works governs to a large extent how healthy and fit you are. When you are cardiovascularly fit, you are functionally younger than your biological age. Research shows that cardiovascular fitness is more important than body weight or body mass index in determining your health and predicting your mortality. Obese individuals with at least moderate cardiovascular fitness have about one-half the rate of cardiovascular disease or all-cause mortality than their normal-weight but unfit peers. In other words, it's better to be overweight and fit than to be thin and out of shape. Cardiovascular endurance is the most important component of physical fitness because the functioning of your cardiovascular system—your heart, arteries, and veins—is so essential to overall health. You cannot live very well or very long without a healthy heart.

Heart disease is the leading cause of death in America. So it pays to make your heart as strong as possible and keep your coronary arteries clear. And cardio workouts do that better than anything else. They clear your coronary arteries, drive your heart rate up, and place a demand on your heart, causing it to respond by becoming stronger. The constant push of oxygen through your blood vessels that occurs when you exercise aerobically is a superb stimulus for waking those vessels up and improving blood flow to all your organs. Cardio workouts increase the amount of hemoglobin inside your red blood cells, which transports oxygen through your blood vessels. The more hemoglobin in your blood, the greater your vessels' oxygen-carrying capability. Cardio workouts also affect your muscles, specifically increasing the amount of mitochondria and enzymes inside of them, making your muscles better consumers of oxygen and better fat-burning machines.

Perhaps the most elegant adaptation your body makes to cardio workouts—especially interval training—is an increase in the size of your heart. The enlargement of the left ventricle of your heart results in a greater stroke volume, which is the amount of blood your heart pumps out with each beat. The larger your left ventricle, the more blood it can hold; the more blood it can hold, the more blood (and oxygen) it can pump. Your cardiovascular fitness and health is largely dictated by your heart's ability to pump blood and oxygen. Make a better heart and you make a healthier person.

Apart from its direct effects on your cardiovascular system, cardio workouts also impact other aspects of your health. They decrease blood pressure, cholesterol, and percent body fat; reduce the symptoms of depression and the risk for certain types of cancer; and increase connections between neurons in your brain, enabling you to think better and more creatively.

There is so much scientific evidence to prove the biological benefits of cardiovascular exercise that it's fair to say that it is the single best thing you can do for your health. If you want to get the most fitness, biggest calorie burn, and most potent health boost out of the least amount of time—like 14 minutes—cardio interval workouts are the most time-efficient workouts you can do. So let's get started.

VO$_2$MAX WORKOUTS

It's Sunday morning. You get out of bed and prepare to go out for a run. You put on your moisture-wicking socks and shirt, lace your shoes, and head out the door. Before you even take your first step, the cortex of your brain stimulates your autonomic nervous system, which causes your blood vessels to constrict and your blood pressure to rise. Within a few strides of your run, you start to breathe faster and deeper. The number of times your heart beats each minute (heart rate) and the volume of blood your heart ejects with each of those beats (stroke volume) both rise to match the greater demand of your muscles for oxygen. More blood flows through your vessels—15 to 20 times more than when you're sitting on your couch. If you keep increasing the pace until you're huffing and puffing like you're going to blow grandma's house down, you'll reach your VO$_2$max, the maximum volume of oxygen your muscles consume per minute.

First measured in humans in the 1920s, VO$_2$max is the single best indicator of your aerobic fitness. Think of VO$_2$max as the size of your aerobic engine. When you exercise at your VO$_2$max, your cardiovascular system is working as hard as it can—your heart rate and stroke volume reach their maximum values, which makes your heart bigger. VO$_2$max intervals are like strength training for your heart.

For the following VO$_2$max interval workouts, all of which take 14 minutes or less to complete, choose your favorite type of cardio exercise (e.g., running, cycling, rowing, or swimming) and alternate periods of high-intensity (hard-effort) exercise and low-intensity (easy-effort) recovery. Keep the recovery intervals active to keep oxygen consumption elevated throughout the workout. This helps you reach your VO$_2$max sooner during each subsequent rep, enabling you to spend more time working at your VO$_2$max intensity during the workout. In addition to using a percentage of your maximum heart rate (HR) as an objective measure of intensity, the workouts also include Rating of Perceived Exertion (RPE) as a subjective measure of intensity. RPE is a rating of how hard the intensity feels and is based on a scale of 1 (easiest) to 10 (hardest). Warm up prior to each workout, starting at a low intensity and progressing to a higher intensity to create a smooth transition from the warm-up to the workout. Begin the workout within a couple of minutes of completing the warm-up.

VO$_2$max 5 x 1

	Duration	RPE	Intensity
Rep #1	1:00	9	>95% max HR
Recovery	2:00	2–3	
Rep #2	1:00	9	>95% max HR
Recovery	2:00	2–3	
Rep #3	1:00	9	>95% max HR
Recovery	2:00	2–3	
Rep #4	1:00	9	>95% max HR
Recovery	2:00	2–3	
Rep #5	1:00	9	>95% max HR
Total Time	13:00		

VO$_2$max 4 x 2

	Duration	RPE	Intensity
Rep #1	2:00	9	>95% max HR
Recovery	2:00	2–3	
Rep #2	2:00	9	>95% max HR
Recovery	2:00	2–3	
Rep #3	2:00	9	>95% max HR
Recovery	2:00	2–3	
Rep #4	2:00	9	>95% max HR
Total Time	14:00		

VO$_2$max 3 x 3

	Duration	RPE	Intensity
Rep #1	3:00	9	>95% max HR
Recovery	2:30	2–3	
Rep #2	3:00	9	>95% max HR
Recovery	2:30	2–3	
Rep #3	3:00	9	>95% max HR
Total Time	14:00		

VO$_2$max 2 x 5

	Duration	RPE	Intensity
Rep #1	5:00	9	>95% max HR
Recovery	4:00	2–3	
Rep #2	5:00	9	>95% max HR
Total Time	14:00		

VO$_2$max Alternating 1–2

	Duration	RPE	Intensity
Rep #1	1:00	9	>95% max HR
Recovery	1:00	2–3	
Rep #2	2:00	9	>95% max HR
Recovery	1:00	2–3	
Rep #3	1:00	9	>95% max HR
Recovery	1:00	2–3	
Rep #4	2:00	9	>95% max HR
Recovery	1:00	2–3	
Rep #5	1:00	9	>95% max HR
Recovery	1:00	2–3	
Rep #6	2:00	9	>95% max HR
Total Time	14:00		

VO$_2$max Ladder

	Duration	RPE	Intensity
Rep #1	1:00	9	>95% max HR
Recovery	1:00	2–3	
Rep #2	2:00	9	>95% max HR
Recovery	2:00	2–3	
Rep #3	2:30	9	>95% max HR
Recovery	2:30	2–3	
Rep #4	3:00	9	>95% max HR
Total Time	14:00		

VO$_2$max Pyramid

	Duration	RPE	Intensity
Rep #1	1:00	9	>95% max HR
Recovery	1:30	2–3	
Rep #2	1:30	9	>95% max HR
Recovery	1:30	2–3	
Rep #3	3:00	9	>95% max HR
Recovery	1:30	2–3	
Rep #4	1:30	9	>95% max HR
Recovery	1:30	2–3	
Rep #5	1:00	9	>95% max HR
Total Time	14:00		

AEROBIC TEMPO WORKOUTS

Tempo workouts are high-end aerobic efforts that are comfortably hard. The intensity of tempo workouts corresponds to an important physiological variable called your acidosis (lactate) threshold, because it marks the onset of acidosis—the drop in pH in your muscles that causes them to become acidic and to fatigue.

When you exercise below the acidosis threshold, the intensity is purely aerobic, but when you exercise above the threshold, it is both aerobic and anaerobic. The higher above your threshold you go, the more anaerobic it becomes and the more you fatigue, in part because of the greater drop in pH in your muscles. The intensity just below and above the threshold is the difference between the effort feeling comfortably hard and uncomfortably hard. Think of the acidosis threshold as the percentage (or fraction) of your VO_2max engine that you can sustain aerobically.

To do the following aerobic tempo workouts, all of which take 14 minutes or less to complete, choose your favorite type of cardio exercise (e.g., running, cycling, rowing, or swimming) and alternate periods of comfortably hard effort and easy-effort recovery. You can do aerobic tempo workouts outside or in a gym. The workouts should feel comfortably hard, with an RPE of 7 to 8 on a scale of 1 to 10, and you should reach about 80 to 85 percent of your maximum heart rate during each rep. Keep the intensity as steady as possible during the workout. To help you hold the rhythm of the workouts, try listening to music with a moderate tempo. Warm up prior to each workout, starting at a low intensity and progressing to a moderate intensity.

Aerobic Tempo 5 x 2

	Duration	RPE	Intensity
Rep #1	2:00	7–8	80–85% max HR
Recovery	:30	2–3	
Rep #2	2:00	7–8	80–85% max HR
Recovery	:30	2–3	
Rep #3	2:00	7–8	80–85% max HR
Recovery	:30	2–3	
Rep #4	2:00	7–8	80–85% max HR
Recovery	:30	2–3	
Rep #5	2:00	7–8	80–85% max HR
Total Time	12:00		

Aerobic Tempo 3 x 4

	Duration	RPE	Intensity
Rep #1	4:00	7–8	80–85% max HR
Recovery	1:00	2–3	
Rep #2	4:00	7–8	80–85% max HR
Recovery	1:00	2–3	
Rep #3	4:00	7–8	80–85% max HR
Total Time	14:00		

Aerobic Tempo 2 x 6

	Duration	RPE	Intensity
Rep #1	6:00	7–8	80–85% max HR
Recovery	2:00	2–3	
Rep #2	6:00	7–8	80–85% max HR
Total Time	14:00		

Continuous Aerobic Tempo

	Duration	RPE	Intensity
Rep #1	14:00	7–8	80–85% max HR
Total Time	14:00		

FARTLEKS

Fartlek, that funny-sounding word known among runners that makes high school girls giggle on the first day of cross-country practice, is a free-form type of high-intensity cardio workout, during which you increase the intensity at different times, when you reach specific landmarks, or simply based on how you feel. Rep duration, intensity, and recovery intervals all vary within the same workout. The workout comes from the Swedish words *fart*, meaning speed, and *lek*, meaning play, and dates back to

1937, when it was developed by Swedish track coach Gösta Holmér to train Sweden's military.

For the following fartleks, all of which take 14 minutes or less to complete, choose your favorite type of cardio exercise (e.g., running, cycling, rowing, or swimming) and alternate periods of hard effort and easy-effort recovery. You can do fartleks outside or in a gym. Listen to your body and increase the intensity based on how you feel, making the hard efforts feel like a 7 to 9 rating of perceived exertion (RPE) on a scale of 1 to 10.

Fartleks are meant to be fun, so have fun with them. Run on a trail or cycle on a bike path around a lake. Warm up prior to each workout, starting at a low intensity and progressing to a moderate intensity.

Classic Fartlek

	Duration	RPE
Reps	7:00	7–9
Recoveries	7:00	4–5
Total Time	**14:00**	

For the Classic Fartlek, which is completely free-form, increase and decrease the intensity whenever you want for however long you want or, if outside, from one landmark to another, for a total of 7 minutes of increased intensity during the workout. If you do the fartlek in the gym on a treadmill, elliptical machine, rowing machine, or bike, increase the intensity one (or more) of three ways:

1) increase only the speed/RPM
2) increase only the grade/resistance
3) increase both the speed/RPM and grade/resistance

1-2-3-2-1 Fartlek

	Duration	RPE
Rep #1	1:00	>7
Recovery	1:00	4–5
Rep #2	2:00	>7
Recovery	1:00	4–5
Rep #3	3:00	>7
Recovery	1:00	4–5
Rep #4	2:00	>7
Recovery	1:00	4–5
Rep #5	1:00	>7
Total Time	13:00	

3-2-2-3 Fartlek

	Duration	RPE
Rep #1	3:00	>7
Recovery	1:00	4–5
Rep #2	2:00	>7
Recovery	1:00	4–5
Rep #3	2:00	>7
Recovery	1:00	4–5
Rep #4	3:00	>7
Total Time	13:00	

4–3–2–1–½ Fartlek

	Duration	RPE
Rep #1	4:00	>7
Recovery	:45	4–5
Rep #2	3:00	>7
Recovery	:45	4–5
Rep #3	2:00	>7
Recovery	:45	4–5
Rep #4	1:00	>7
Recovery	:45	4–5
Rep #5	:30	>7
Total Time	**13:30**	

TREADMILL HILL INTERVALS

Hill intervals are great workouts for your cardiovascular and muscular systems because of the demand on the heart and skeletal muscles. Running up a hill increases your muscles' demand for oxygen. It also sculpts your legs and butt and increases leg muscle power.

You can modify the workouts by walking up the hills instead of running. Exaggerate your arm swing, lean into the hill from your ankles (not from your waist), and focus on pushing off the treadmill belt with the ball of your foot and quickly pulling your knee to the front of your body for the next step.

You can also do these workouts outside, although it's easier to manipulate the grade of the hill on a treadmill. These workouts are intense, so warm up prior to each workout, starting at a low intensity and progressing to a higher intensity so that you create a smooth transition from the warm-up to the workout. Begin the workout within a couple of minutes of completing the warm-up.

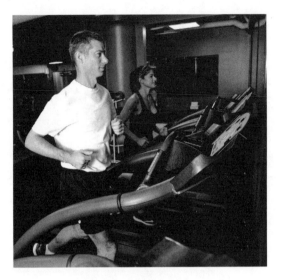

Treadmill Hill Pyramid 1

	Duration	Grade	RPE	Intensity
Rep #1	1:00	2%	8	85–90% max HR
Recovery	1:00	0%	2–3	
Rep #2	1:00	4%	8	85–90% max HR
Recovery	1:00	0%	2–3	
Rep #3	1:00	6%	8.5	85–90% max HR
Recovery	1:00	0%	2–3	
Rep #4	1:00	8%	9	>90% max HR
Recovery	1:00	0%	2–3	
Rep #5	1:00	6%	8.5	85–90% max HR
Recovery	1:00	0%	2–3	
Rep #6	1:00	4%	8	85–90% max HR
Recovery	1:00	0%	2–3	
Rep #7	1:00	2%	8	85–90% max HR
Total Time	13:00			

Use the same workout speed for each rep and the same recovery speed for each recovery interval. For the reps, choose a speed that is challenging. For the recovery intervals, decrease the speed to a slow jog that enables you to recover before the next rep.

Treadmill Hill Pyramid 2

	Duration	Grade	Speed	RPE	Intensity
Rep #1	1:00	2%	Starting speed	8	85–90% max HR
Recovery	1:00	0%	Half starting speed	2–3	
Rep #2	1:00	4%	Starting speed - 0.5 mph	8	85–90% max HR
Recovery	1:00	0%	Half starting speed	2–3	
Rep #3	1:00	6%	Starting speed - 1.0 mph	8.5	85–90% max HR
Recovery	1:00	0%	Half starting speed	2–3	
Rep #4	1:00	8%	Starting speed - 1.5 mph	9	>90% max HR
Recovery	1:00	0%	Half starting speed	2–3	
Rep #5	1:00	6%	Starting speed - 1.0 mph	8.5	85–90% max HR
Recovery	1:00	0%	Half starting speed	2–3	
Rep #6	1:00	4%	Starting speed - 0.5 mph	8	85–90% max HR
Recovery	1:00	0%	Half starting speed	2–3	
Rep #7	1:00	2%	Starting speed	8	85–90% max HR
Total Time	13:00				

Choose a starting speed that is challenging but doable. Speed decreases by 0.5 mph on ascending reps and increases by 0.5 mph on descending reps. For the recovery intervals, decrease the speed to half of the starting speed or to as slow as you need to recover before the next rep.

Treadmill Hill Ladder

	Duration	Grade	RPE	Intensity
Rep #1	1:00	2%	8	85–90% max HR
Recovery	1:00	0%	2–3	
Rep #2	1:00	4%	8	85–90% max HR
Recovery	1:00	0%	2–3	
Rep #3	1:00	6%	8.5	85–90% max HR
Recovery	1:00	0%	2–3	
Rep #4	1:00	8%	9	>90% max HR
Recovery	1:00	0%	2–3	
Rep #5	1:00	10%	9	>90% max HR
Recovery	1:00	0%	2–3	
Rep #6	1:00	12%	9	>90% max HR
Recovery	1:00	0%	2–3	
Rep #7	1:00	14%	9	>90% max HR
Total Time	13:00			

Use the same workout speed for each rep and the same recovery speed for each recovery interval. For the reps, choose a speed that is challenging. For the recovery intervals, decrease the speed to a slow jog that enables you to recover before the next rep.

Treadmill Triple 3 Hills
3 Reps, 3 Minutes, 3% Grade

	Duration	Grade	RPE	Intensity
Rep #1	3:00	3%	9	>90% max HR
Recovery	2:00	0%	2–3	
Rep #2	3:00	3%	9	>90% max HR
Recovery	2:00	0%	2–3	
Rep #3	3:00	3%	9	>90% max HR
Total Time	13:00			

Use the same workout speed for each rep and the same recovery speed for each recovery interval. For the reps, choose a speed that is challenging. For the recovery intervals, decrease the speed to a slow jog that enables you to recover before the next rep.

CHAPTER 2

SPRINT WORKOUTS

If you watch fourth graders run, you'll notice that they run fast for a brief period, stop for an interval to catch their breath, and run fast again for a brief period. They don't instinctively run slowly for long periods of time without stopping. Fourth graders like to run fast. From the time I ran the 50-yard dash as part of the Presidential Physical Fitness Test in fourth grade, I knew that I, too, liked to run fast.

When I was a kid, my athletic idol was Carl Lewis. After watching him win four gold medals at the 1984 Olympics, I would go outside and sprint as fast as I could down the sidewalk in front of my mother's house, wearing an old pair of Puma spikes I had dug out of the bottom of my closet. I have always loved speed. And so sprinting is how I became a competitive runner, running the 100-meter and 400-meter races on my middle school track team.

Sprinting allows you to let go, to feel powerful and strong, and to recruit fast-twitch muscle fibers that are dormant the rest of the day. The funny thing about muscle fibers is that their recruitment is dictated by what we need to perform the task. If you never sprint, you don't recruit the fast-twitch fibers. When you sprint, however, you recruit nearly everything in your muscles' arsenal—slow-twitch *and* fast-twitch fibers. Use it or lose it, as the saying goes.

By recruiting fast-twitch muscle fibers, sprinting increases your muscle power and makes you very fit. There's nothing quite like sprint workouts to make your legs, glutes, and core tight and toned. There's a reason why sprinters have attractive bodies. Because of their potent effect on your fitness and muscle power, sprint workouts also make your other workouts feel easier, which enables you to challenge yourself at a harder level during other workouts and burn even more calories. Train your inner sprinter, and watch your body change.

For the following sprint interval workouts, all of which take 14 minutes or less to complete, choose your favorite type of cardio exercise (e.g., running, cycling, rowing, or swimming), and alternate periods of fast effort and easy-effort recovery. Fast should feel like you are nearly sprinting, but don't go so fast that you cannot repeat the same intensity after the short recovery. Keep the recovery intervals active. These workouts are intense, so warm up prior to each workout, starting at a low intensity and progressing to a higher intensity so that you create a smooth transition from the warm-up to the workout. For example, whichever type of exercise you choose for the workout, do it for 10 minutes at a low intensity to warm up, increasing the intensity a little each minute or two. After 10 minutes, do a few bursts of exercise at a high intensity for 5 to 10 seconds to prime your muscles for the intensity of the workout. Take enough time to recover between each burst since these bursts are not part of the workout and shouldn't cause fatigue; they are only meant to prepare your body for the intensity of the workout. Begin the workout within a couple of minutes of completing the warm-up.

Sprint 10 x 10

	Duration	RPE	Intensity
Rep #1	:10	10	Fast
Recovery	:30	2–3	
Rep #2	:10	10	Fast
Recovery	:30	2–3	
Rep #3	:10	10	Fast
Recovery	:30	2–3	
Rep #4	:10	10	Fast
Recovery	:30	2–3	
Rep #5	:10	10	Fast

Recovery	:30	2–3	
Rep #6	:10	10	Fast
Recovery	:30	2–3	
Rep #7	:10	10	Fast
Recovery	:30	2–3	
Rep #8	:10	10	Fast
Recovery	:30	2–3	
Rep #9	:10	10	Fast
Recovery	:30	2–3	
Rep #10	:10	10	Fast
Total Time	**6:10**		

Sprint 10 x 20

	Duration	RPE	Intensity
Rep #1	:20	9	Fast
Recovery	1:00	2–3	
Rep #2	:20	9	Fast
Recovery	1:00	2–3	
Rep #3	:20	9	Fast
Recovery	1:00	2–3	
Rep #4	:20	9	Fast
Recovery	1:00	2–3	
Rep #5	:20	9	Fast
Recovery	1:00	2–3	
Rep #6	:20	9	Fast
Recovery	1:00	2–3	
Rep #7	:20	9	Fast
Recovery	1:00	2–3	
Rep #8	:20	9	Fast
Recovery	1:00	2–3	
Rep #9	:20	9	Fast
Recovery	1:00	2–3	
Rep #10	:20	9	Fast
Total Time	**12:20**		

Sprint 10 x 30

	Duration	RPE	Intensity
Rep #1	:30	9	Fast
Recovery	1:00	2–3	
Rep #2	:30	9	Fast
Recovery	1:00	2–3	
Rep #3	:30	9	Fast
Recovery	1:00	2–3	
Rep #4	:30	9	Fast
Recovery	1:00	2–3	
Rep #5	:30	9	Fast
Recovery	1:00	2–3	
Rep #6	:30	9	Fast
Recovery	1:00	2–3	
Rep #7	:30	9	Fast
Recovery	1:00	2–3	
Rep #8	:30	9	Fast
Recovery	1:00	2–3	
Rep #9	:30	9	Fast
Recovery	1:00	2–3	
Rep #10	:30	9	Fast
Total Time	14:00		

Sprint 5 x 1

	Duration	RPE	Intensity
Rep #1	1:00	9	Fast
Recovery	2:00	2–3	
Rep #2	1:00	9	Fast
Recovery	2:00	2–3	
Rep #3	1:00	9	Fast
Recovery	2:00	2–3	
Rep #4	1:00	9	Fast
Recovery	2:00	2–3	
Rep #5	1:00	9	Fast
Total Time	13:00		

Sprint Ladder

	Duration	RPE	Intensity
Set #1			
Rep #1	:10	9	Fast
Recovery	:20	2–3	
Rep #2	:20	9	Fast
Recovery	:40	2–3	
Rep #3	:30	9	Fast
Recovery	1:00	2–3	
Rep #4	:40	9	Fast
Recovery	1:20	2–3	
Rep #5	:50	9	Fast
Recovery	1:40	2–3	
Set #2			
Rep #1	:10	9	Fast
Recovery	:20	2–3	
Rep #2	:20	9	Fast
Recovery	:40	2–3	
Rep #3	:30	9	Fast
Recovery	1:00	2–3	
Rep #4	:40	9	Fast
Recovery	1:20	2–3	
Rep #5	:50	9	Fast
Total Time	**13:20**		

Sprint Pyramid

	Duration	RPE	Intensity
Rep #1	:10	9	Fast
Recovery	:20	2–3	
Rep #2	:20	9	Fast
Recovery	:40	2–3	
Rep #3	:30	9	Fast
Recovery	1:00	2–3	
Rep #4	:40	9	Fast
Recovery	1:20	2–3	
Rep #5	:50	9	Fast
Recovery	1:40	2–3	
Rep #6	:40	9	Fast
Recovery	1:20	2–3	
Rep #7	:30	9	Fast
Recovery	1:00	2–3	
Rep #8	:20	9	Fast
Recovery	:40	2–3	
Rep #9	:10	9	Fast
Total Time	**12:10**		

True Tabata

	Duration	RPE	Intensity
Rep #1	:20	10	Nearly all-out
Recovery	:10	2	
Rep #2	:20	10	Nearly all-out
Recovery	:10	2	
Rep #3	:20	10	Nearly all-out
Recovery	:10	2	
Rep #4	:20	10	Nearly all-out
Recovery	:10	2	
Rep #5	:20	10	Nearly all-out
Recovery	:10	2	
Rep #6	:20	10	Nearly all-out
Recovery	:10	2	
Rep #7	:20	10	Nearly all-out
Recovery	:10	2	
Rep #8	:20	10	Nearly all-out
Total Time	3:50		

Do this workout on a stationary bike and sprint nearly as fast as you can for each 20-second rep. In Japanese scientist Dr. Izumi Tabata's original research study published in 1996 (spin-offs of which have become a popular method of fitness training), subjects cycled 7 to 8 reps at 170% VO_2max, which was determined from previous VO_2max tests in their laboratory, and they did that workout five times per week for six weeks. Don't try that at home!

CHAPTER 3

MUSCULAR ENDURANCE WORKOUTS

When I was in eighth grade, I did 24 chin-ups to break the school record. I still have the certificate of achievement from the school's principal proudly displayed on my wall. I still brag about the accomplishment to others. It doesn't matter that it was so many years ago or that some tough kid has probably come along since to break my record. At the time, I had the strongest biceps and best-looking arms in middle school. I used chin-ups to show off to the girls in my class. I attached a chin-up bar to my bedroom doorframe so I could train at home. I did chin-ups every day. My mother even surprised me the day I broke the record with a cake featuring a chin-up bar iced on it in chocolate. I was a hero. What I learned from chin-ups is that there is more than one way to train a muscle (and it's a great way to get girls' attention!).

To increase muscular endurance and get shapely muscles, muscles need to contract against a low to moderate resistance—60 to 80 percent of the maximum you can lift just once—with short recovery intervals between sets. To improve endurance, what matters is the amount of time the muscles are under tension. All of the workouts in this chapter are designed to be completed in 14 minutes or less.

MACHINE WORKOUTS

Upper Body 1: Back & Biceps

Exercise	Sets	Reps	Intensity (% 1 rep max or RPE)	Recovery
Chin-Ups	3–4	15–20	70–75%	:30
Seated Cable Row	3–4	15–20	70–75%	:30
Biceps Preacher Curls	3–4	15–20	70–75%	:30

EXERCISE INSTRUCTIONS

Chin-Ups

Stand on the platform of a weight-assisted chin-up machine. Grab the handles of the machine above your head with an underhand grip [1]. Pull yourself up until your chin reaches the height of your hands [2]. Lower yourself down to the starting position and repeat for the prescribed number of reps.

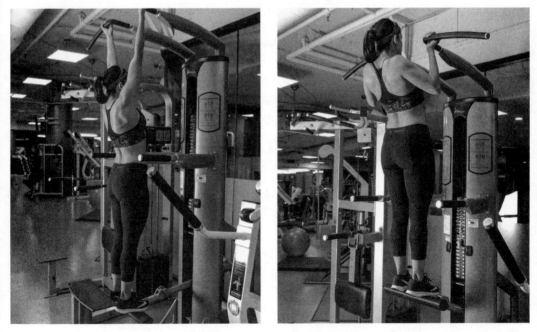

1   2

Seated Cable Row

Sit down on the machine and place your feet on the front platform with your knees slightly bent. Lean forward to grab the handles of the bar (use a V-bar that will keep your hands facing each other). Scoot back on the seat and pull the bar back with arms extended until your hips are at a 90-degree angle to your torso and your back is straight [1]. Using your back muscles, pull the handles of the bar toward your torso [2]. Slowly return to the starting position to lower the weight and repeat for the prescribed number of reps.

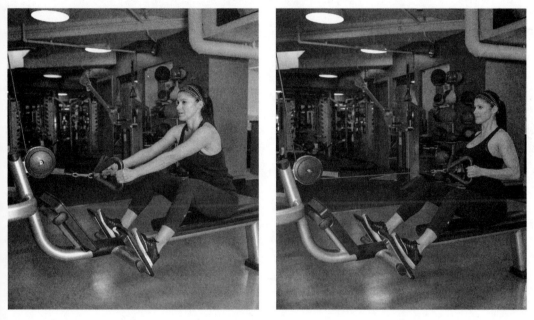

1   2

Biceps Preacher Curls

Sit on the seat of the machine and adjust the seat height so that you can comfortably extend your arms on the pad and your elbows are in line with the pivot point of the machine. Lay the back of your arms on the pad and grab the handles with an underhand grip [1]. Lift the weight by flexing your elbows, pulling your hands toward your shoulders [2]. Slowly return to the starting position to lower the weight and repeat for the prescribed number of reps.

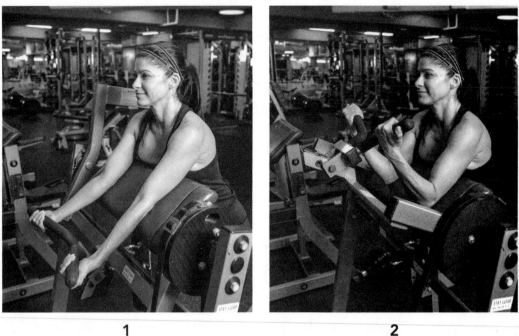

1   2

Upper Body 2: Chest, Shoulders, & Triceps

Exercise	Sets	Reps	Intensity (% 1 rep max or RPE)	Recovery
Chest Press	3–4	15–20	70–75%	:30
Shoulder Press	3–4	15–20	70–75%	:30
Triceps Pressdown	3–4	15–20	70–75%	:30

EXERCISE INSTRUCTIONS

Chest Press

Sit with your back straight and flat against the back pad of the machine with feet flat on the floor. Grip the handles near your chest with an overhand grip [1]. Extend your arms to push the handles forward and up to lift the weight [2]. Slowly return to the starting position to lower the weight and repeat for the prescribed number of reps.

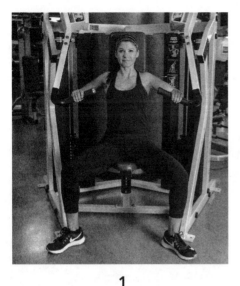
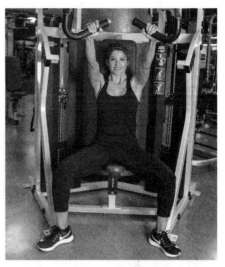

1   2

Shoulder Press

Sit down on the machine's seat with your back straight against the back pad. Adjust the seat height so that when you grab the handles, your hands are in line with your shoulders [1]. Push upward to lift the weight until your arms are fully extended [2]. Slowly return to the starting position to lower the weight and repeat for the prescribed number of reps.

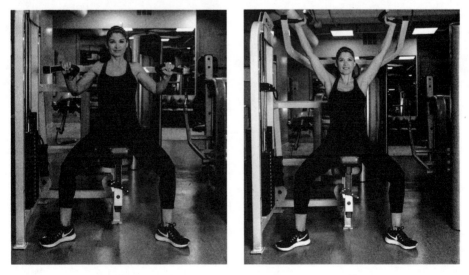

1   2

Triceps Pressdown

Attach a straight bar to a high pulley and grab the bar, using an overhand grip with your hands slightly less than shoulder-width apart. Stand with feet shoulder-width apart and your torso straight. Hold your upper arms close to your body with your elbows in to your sides and pointing down toward the floor [1]. Using your triceps, push the bar down until your arms are fully extended. Keep your upper arms stationary throughout the movement and hold them next to your torso [2]. Slowly return to the starting position to lower the weight and repeat for the prescribed number of reps.

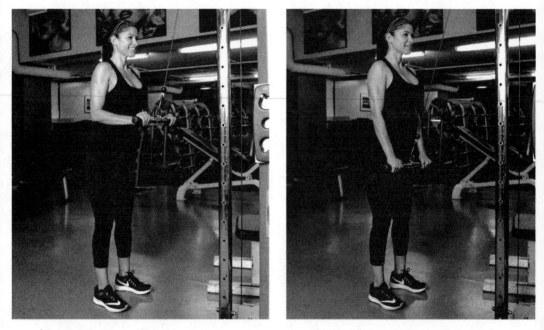

1   2

Lower Body 1: Quads & Calves

Exercise	Sets	Reps	Intensity (% 1 rep max or RPE)	Recovery
Squats (Smith machine)	3–4	15–20	70–75%	:30
Calf Press	3–4	15–20	70–75%	:30
Leg Press	3–4	15–20	70–75%	:30

EXERCISE INSTRUCTIONS

Squats (Smith machine)

Set the bar on the Smith machine to the height of your shoulders. Place any extra weight on the bar that you need to meet the prescribed intensity. With feet shoulder-width or slightly greater than shoulder-width apart, stand in front of the barbell. Place the barbell across the back of your shoulders below your neck and grab the barbell from behind with a grip slightly greater than shoulder-width. Lift the barbell from the rack so it rests on your shoulders and upper back [1]. Keeping your back straight, bend your knees and squat down until your thighs are parallel to the floor. Move your hips back as if you're going to sit in a chair [2]. Push against the floor to return to the starting position and repeat for the prescribed number of reps.

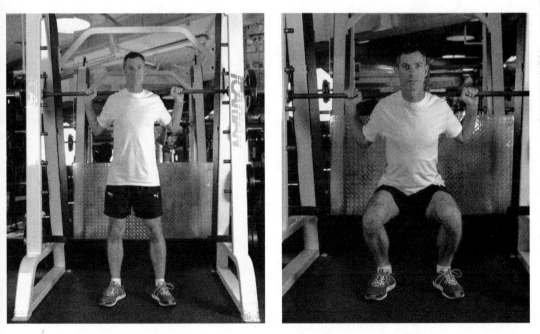

1   **2**

Calf Press

Sit on the seat of a seated calf press machine and place your toes and the balls of your feet on the platform in front of you with your feet shoulder-width apart, legs slightly bent, and your back against the seat cushion. Grab the side handles of the machine for support [1]. Push against the platform with the balls of your feet to lift the weight [2]. Slowly return to the starting position and repeat for the prescribed number of reps.

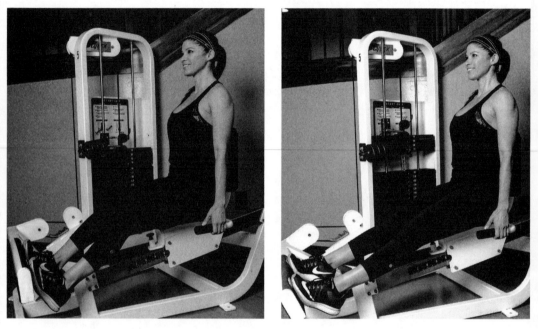

1   2

Leg Press

Sit on the leg press machine with your feet shoulder-width apart on the platform and your back flat against the back pad. Adjust the seat position so that your knees are bent at 90 degrees. Grab the side handles for support [1]. Lift the weight by pressing your feet against the platform and straightening your legs until just before your legs are completely straight [2]. Throughout the motion, keep your legs parallel to one another. Slowly return to the starting position to lower the weight and repeat for the prescribed number of reps.

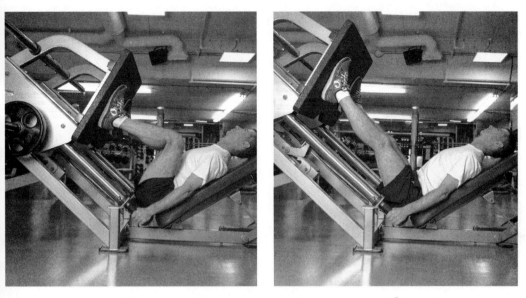

1   2

Lower Body 2: Hamstrings, Glutes, & Inner Thighs

Exercise	Sets	Reps	Intensity (% 1 rep max or RPE)	Recovery
Leg Curl	3–4	15–20	70–75%	:30
Hip Extension	3–4	15–20	70–75%	:30
Low-Cable Deadlift	3–4	15–20	70–75%	:30

EXERCISE INSTRUCTIONS

Leg Curl

Lie facedown on the leg curl machine with your hips flat against the bench, your legs straight, and the leg pad on the back of your legs, just below your calves. Adjust the length of the lever and your position on the pad so that when you lie down, your knees are in line with the pivot point of the machine. Grab the handles of the machine for support [1]. Curl your legs up until your heels come close to your butt [2]. Slowly return to the starting position to lower the weight and repeat for the prescribed number of reps.

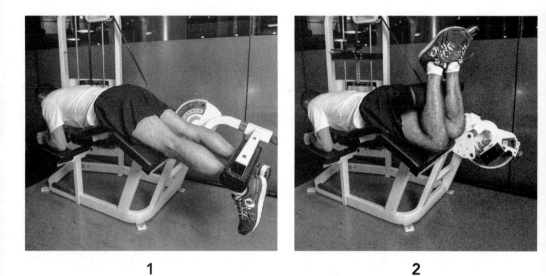

1 2

Hip Extension

Hook an ankle cuff to a low cable pulley and attach the cuff to your ankle. Stand about two feet from the machine, lean slightly forward, and grab the frame for support [1]. Squeeze your glutes and extend the cuffed leg backward, keeping the leg straight [2]. Slowly return to the starting position and repeat for the prescribed number of reps before switching to the other leg.

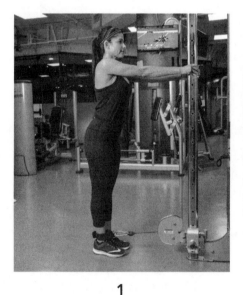
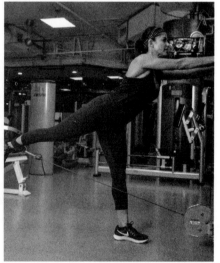

1 2

Low-Cable Deadlift

Attach a straight bar to the cable machine and set it to the lowest setting. Grab the bar with an overhand, shoulder-width grip and step back about two steps. Stand with your feet shoulder-width apart, legs straight or slightly bent, and bend over from your waist with your back straight [1]. Lift the bar by raising your torso to stand up straight, keeping your legs and back straight [2]. Slowly lower the bar to the starting position and repeat for the prescribed number of reps.

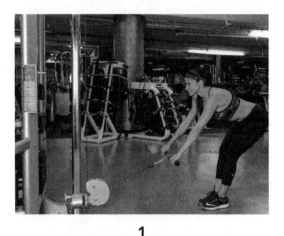

1

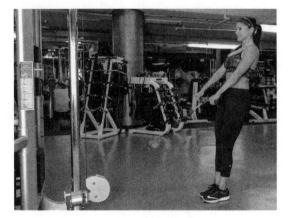

2

Total Body Machine Workout

Exercise	Sets	Reps	Intensity (% 1 rep max or RPE)
Leg Press	1	as many as possible	70–75%
Seated Cable Row	1	as many as possible	70–75%
Leg Curl	1	as many as possible	70–75%
Chest Press	1	as many as possible	70–75%
Hip Extension	1	as many as possible	70–75%
Shoulder Press	1	as many as possible	70–75%
Calf Press	1	as many as possible	70–75%
Biceps Preacher Curls	1	as many as possible	70–75%

Exercises alternate between lower body and upper body and progress from bigger muscles to smaller muscles. Move immediately from one exercise to the next.

EXERCISE INSTRUCTIONS

Leg Press

Sit on the leg press machine with your feet shoulder-width apart on the platform and your back flat against the back pad. Adjust the seat position so that your knees are bent at 90 degrees. Grab the side handles for support [1]. Lift the weight by pressing your feet against the platform and straightening your legs until just before your legs are completely straight [2]. Throughout the motion, keep your legs parallel to one another. Slowly return to the starting position to lower the weight and repeat for the prescribed number of reps.

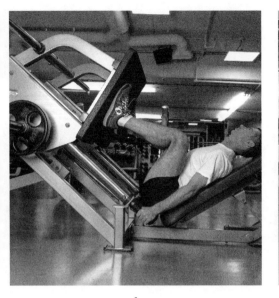

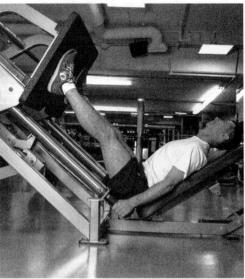

1   2

Seated Cable Row

Sit down on the machine and place your feet on the front platform with your knees slightly bent. Lean forward to grab the handles of the bar (use a V-bar that will keep your hands facing each other). Scoot back on the seat and pull the bar back with arms extended until your hips are at a 90-degree angle to your torso and your back is straight [1]. Using your back muscles, pull the handles of the bar toward your torso [2]. Slowly return to the starting position to lower the weight and repeat for the prescribed number of reps.

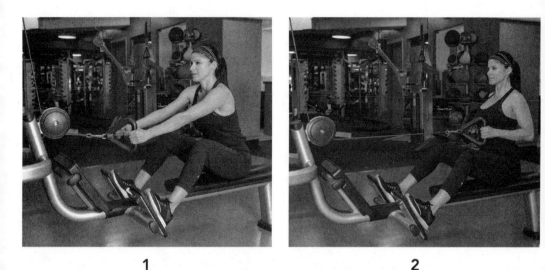

1   2

Leg Curl

Lie facedown on the leg curl machine with your hips flat against the bench, your legs straight, and the leg pad on the back of your legs, just below your calves. Adjust the length of the lever and your position on the pad so that when you lie down, your knees are in line with the pivot point of the machine. Grab the handles of the machine for support [1]. Curl your legs up until your heels come close to your butt [2]. Slowly return to the starting position to lower the weight and repeat for the prescribed number of reps.

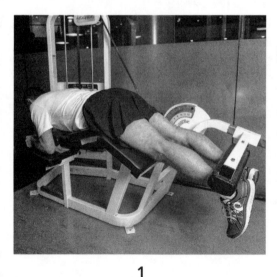

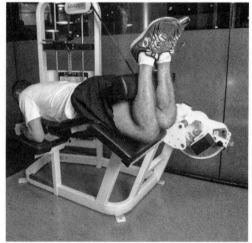

1   2

Chest Press

Sit with your back straight and flat against the back pad of the machine with feet flat on the floor. Grip the handles near your chest with an overhand grip [1]. Extend your arms to push the handles forward and up to lift the weight [2]. Slowly return to the starting position to lower the weight and repeat for the prescribed number of reps.

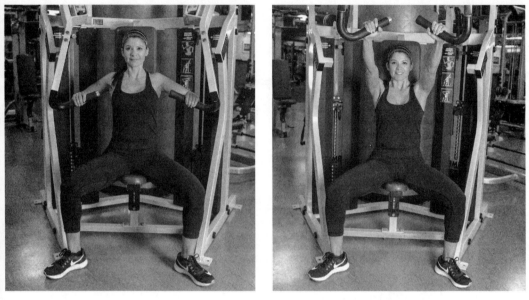

1   2

Hip Extension

Hook an ankle cuff to a low cable pulley and attach the cuff to your ankle. Stand about two feet from the machine, lean slightly forward, and grab the frame for support [1]. Squeeze your glutes and extend the cuffed leg backward, keeping the leg straight [2]. Slowly return to the starting position and repeat for the prescribed number of reps before switching to the other leg.

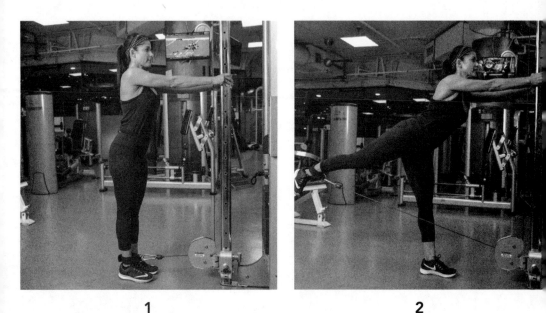

| 1 | 2 |

Shoulder Press

Sit down on the machine's seat with your back straight against the back pad. Adjust the seat height so that when you grab the handles, your hands are in line with your shoulders [1]. Push upward to lift the weight until your arms are fully extended [2]. Slowly return to the starting position to lower the weight and repeat for the prescribed number of reps.

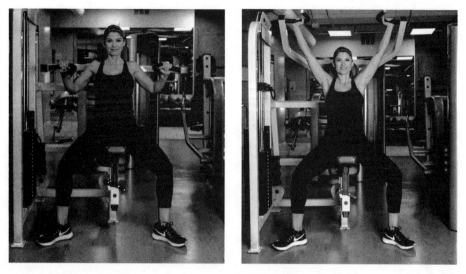

1   2

Calf Press

Sit on the seat of a seated calf press machine and place your toes and the balls of your feet on the platform in front of you with your feet shoulder-width apart, legs slightly bent, and your back against the seat cushion. Grab the side handles of the machine for support [1]. Push against the platform with the balls of your feet to lift the weight [2]. Slowly return to the starting position and repeat for the prescribed number of reps.

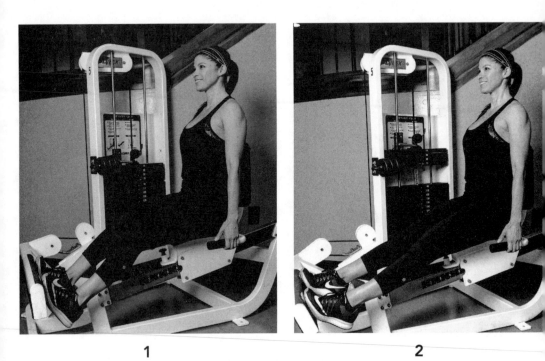

1   2

Biceps Preacher Curls

Sit on the seat of the machine and adjust the seat height so that you can comfortably extend your arms on the pad and your elbows are in line with the pivot point of the machine. Lay the back of your arms on the pad and grab the handles with an underhand grip [1]. Lift the weight by flexing your elbows, pulling your hands toward your shoulders [2]. Slowly return to the starting position to lower the weight and repeat for the prescribed number of reps.

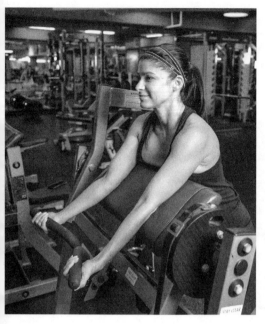

1

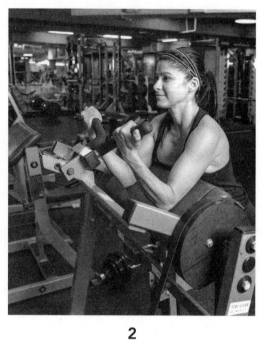

2

DUMBBELL WORKOUTS

Upper Body 1: Back & Biceps

Exercise	Sets	Reps	Intensity (% 1 rep max or RPE)	Recovery
Dumbbell Row	3–4	15–20	70–75%	:30
Dumbbell Reverse Flys	3–4	15–20	70–75%	:30
Dumbbell Biceps Curls	3–4	15–20	70–75%	:30

EXERCISE INSTRUCTIONS

Dumbbell Row

Stand with feet shoulder-width apart with knees slightly bent and hold a dumbbell in each hand with palms facing each other. Keeping your back straight, bend over at the waist until your back is almost parallel to the floor. The dumbbells should hang directly in front of you as your arms hang perpendicular to the floor and your torso [1]. While keeping your torso stationary, use your shoulder muscles to lift the dumbbells, keeping your elbows close to your body [2]. Slowly lower the dumbbells to the starting position and repeat for the prescribed number of reps.

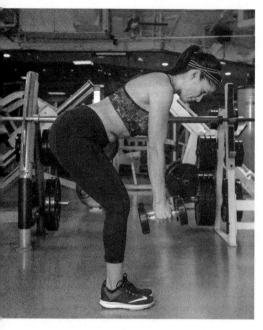 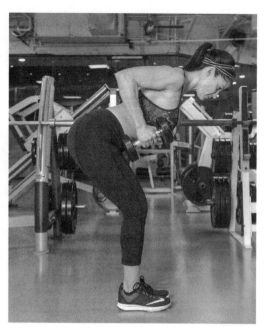

1 **2**

Dumbbell Reverse Flys

Grab a dumbbell in each hand with an overhand grip and palms facing each other and stand with feet shoulder-width apart. Slightly bend your knees and lean forward from your hips with your back straight. Hold the dumbbells with your arms slightly bent [1]. Raise your arms out to your sides like a fly opening its wings until your elbows are slightly higher than your shoulders [2]. Lower the dumbbells to the starting position and repeat for the prescribed number of reps. You can also do this exercise on an incline bench with your torso flat against the bench [3 & 4].

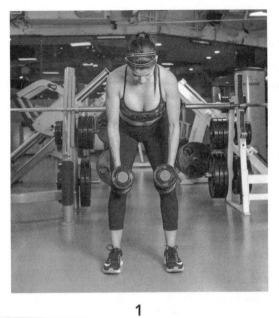

1

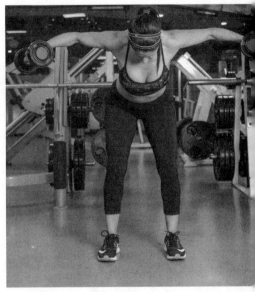

2

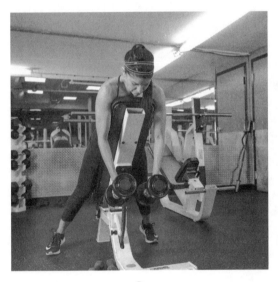

3

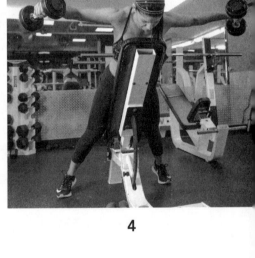

4

14-MINUTE METABOLIC WORKOUTS

Dumbbell Biceps Curls

Stand with feet shoulder-width apart and your back straight. Hold a dumbbell in each hand with your arms by your sides. Keep your elbows close to your body [1]. Lift the dumbbells by bending your elbows and rotate your hands so that your palms face up as the dumbbells reach your shoulders [2]. Lower the dumbbells to the starting position and repeat for the prescribed number of reps.

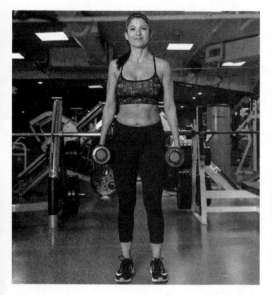

1

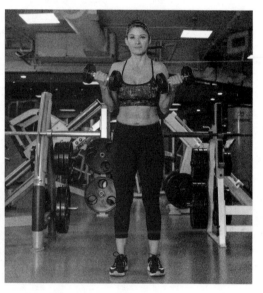

2

Upper Body 2: Chest, Shoulders, & Triceps

Exercise	Sets	Reps	Intensity (% 1 rep max or RPE)	Recovery
Dumbbell Chest Press	3–4	15–20	70–75%	:30
Dumbbell Overhead Press	3–4	15–20	70–75%	:30
Dumbbell Triceps Kickback	3–4	15–20	70–75%	:30

Dumbbell Chest Press

Grab a dumbbell in each hand with an overhand grip and lie on your back on a flat bench with your feet flat on the floor. Hold the dumbbells slightly greater than shoulder-width apart at the level of your chest with the palms of your hands facing each other and your elbows bent at 90 degrees with upper arms parallel to the floor [1]. In one curved motion, push the dumbbells upward by straightening your arms and bring the dumbbells in toward the midline of your chest while rotating your hands so that your palms face away from you as the ends of the dumbbells meet [2]. Lower the dumbbells back along the same arc to the level of your chest and repeat for the prescribed number of reps.

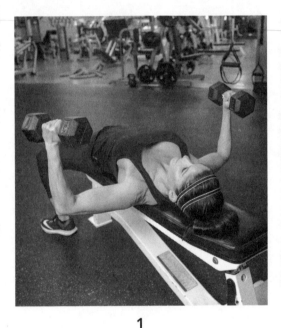

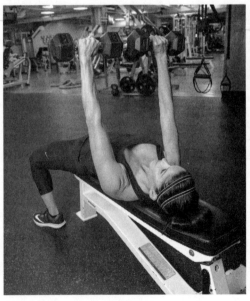

1   2

Dumbbell Overhead Press

Stand with feet shoulder-width apart. Hold a dumbbell in each hand with elbows bent at 90 degrees and pointing down and palms facing forward [1]. Press the dumbbells up and in together over your head [2]. Lower the dumbbells back along the same arc to the starting position, keeping the weight balanced over your elbows, and repeat for the prescribed number of reps.

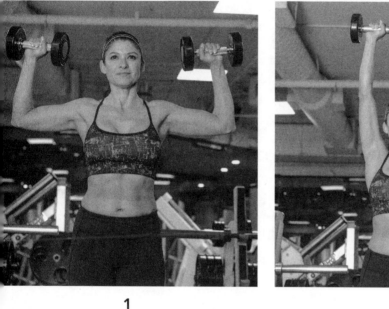

1   2

Dumbbell Triceps Kickback

Kneel on a bench with your left leg and place your left arm on the bench for support. Hold a dumbbell in your right hand with your upper arm parallel to the floor and your elbow bent at 90 degrees [1]. Extend your arm at the elbow until your arm is straight. Only your forearm should move [2]. Slowly return to the starting position and repeat for the prescribed number of reps before switching to the left arm.

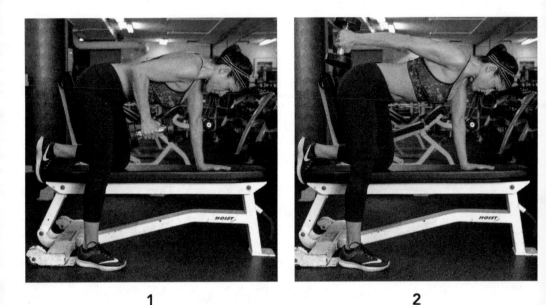

1   2

Lower Body 1: Quads & Calves

Exercise	Sets	Reps	Intensity (% 1 rep max or RPE)	Recovery
Dumbbell Squats	3–4	15–20	70–75%	:30
Dumbbell Calf Raises	3–4	15–20	70–75%	:30
Dumbbell Step-Ups	3–4	15–20	70–75%	:30

EXERCISE INSTRUCTIONS

Dumbbell Squats

Stand with feet shoulder-width or slightly wider than shoulder-width apart with a dumbbell in each hand and arms fully extended with palms facing the side of your legs [1]. Keeping your back straight, bend your knees and squat down until your thighs are parallel to the floor. Move your hips back as if you're going to sit in a chair [2]. Push against the floor to return to the starting position and repeat for the prescribed number of reps.

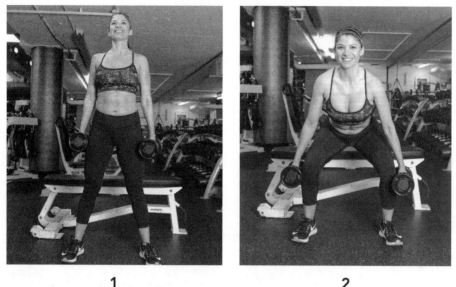

1   2

Dumbbell Calf Raises

Hold a dumbbell in each hand and stand with legs together, with one foot off the ground [1]. With the other foot, push against the ground with the ball of your foot to raise yourself up [2]. Slowly return to the starting position and repeat for the prescribed number of reps.

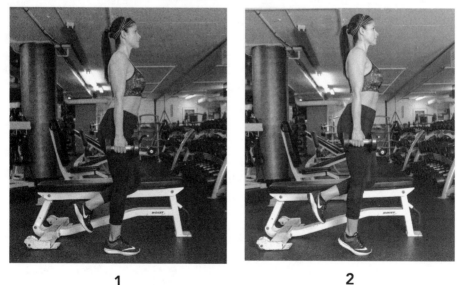

1   2

Dumbbell Step-Ups

Stand behind a bench or other elevated platform with a dumbbell in each hand and your palms facing the side of your legs [1]. Step up onto the bench with your right leg [2] and then place your left foot on the bench [3]. Step down with your left leg to return to the starting position and repeat for the prescribed number of reps before switching to leading with the left leg.

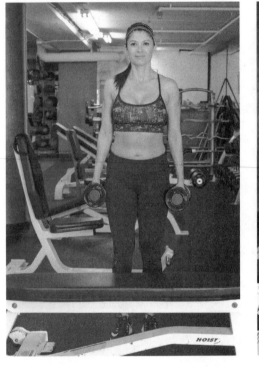

1

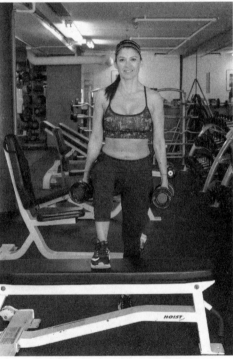

2

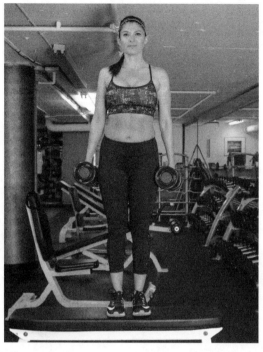

3

Lower Body 2: Hamstrings, Glutes, & Inner Thighs

Exercise	Sets	Reps	Intensity (% 1 rep max or RPE)	Recovery
Dumbbell Deadlift	3–4	15–20	70–75%	:30
Dumbbell Side Lunges	3–4	15–20	70–75%	:30
Dumbbell Plié Squats	3–4	15–20	70–75%	:30

EXERCISE INSTRUCTIONS

Dumbbell Deadlift

Hold a dumbbell in each hand by your sides at arm's length and stand with your feet shoulder-width apart [1]. Keeping your back and legs straight, bend over at the waist to lower the dumbbells until your back is parallel to the floor. As you bend over, you should feel a stretch in your hamstrings [2]. Keeping your back and legs straight, stand upright to return to the starting position and repeat for the prescribed number of reps.

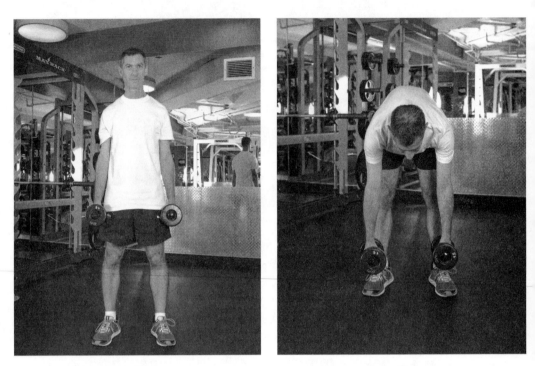

1   2

Dumbbell Side Lunges

Hold a dumbbell in each hand in front of you, with your palms facing each other, and stand with your feet shoulder-width apart [1]. Take a big lateral step out to your left side and lower yourself into a squat, keeping your right leg straight [2]. Push back up with your left leg to return to the starting position and repeat for the prescribed number of reps before switching to the right leg.

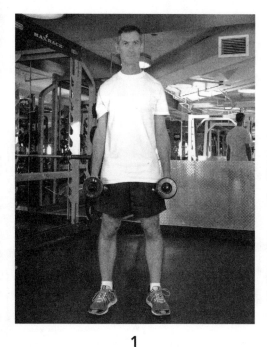 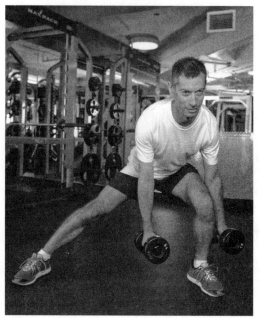

1   2

Dumbbell Plié Squats

Stand with feet slightly greater than shoulder-width apart and toes turned out about 45 degrees. Hold a dumbbell vertically with both hands between your legs [1]. Keeping your back straight, squat down until your thighs are parallel to the floor [2]. Push through your feet to stand up to return to the starting position and repeat for the prescribed number of reps.

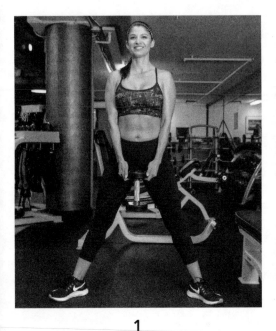

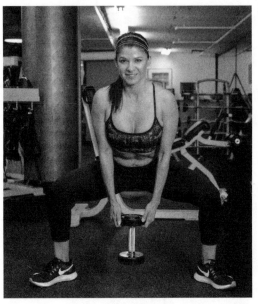

1   2

Total Body Dumbbell Workout

Exercise	Sets	Reps	Intensity (% 1 rep max or RPE)
Dumbbell Plié Squats	1	as many as possible	70–75%
Dumbbell Chest Press	1	as many as possible	70–75%
Dumbbell Lunges	1	as many as possible	70–75%
Dumbbell Reverse Flys	1	as many as possible	70–75%
Dumbbell Deadlift	1	as many as possible	70–75%
Dumbbell Row	1	as many as possible	70–75%
Dumbbell Calf Raises	1	as many as possible	70–75%
Dumbbell Biceps Curls	1	as many as possible	70–75%

Exercises alternate between lower body and upper body and progress from bigger muscles to smaller muscles. Move immediately from one exercise to the next.

Dumbbell Plié Squats

Stand with feet slightly greater than shoulder-width apart and toes turned out about 45 degrees. Hold a dumbbell vertically with both hands between your legs [1]. Keeping your back straight, squat down until your thighs are parallel to the floor [2]. Push through your feet to stand up to return to the starting position and repeat for the prescribed number of reps.

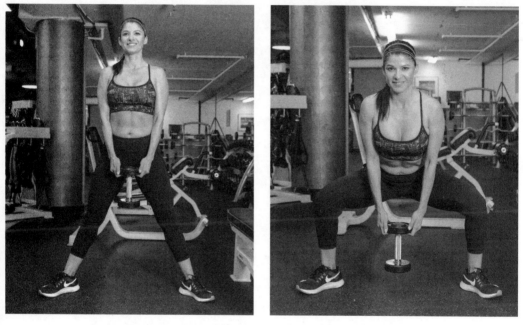

1   2

Dumbbell Chest Press

Grab a dumbbell in each hand with an overhand grip and lie on your back on a flat bench with your feet flat on the floor. Hold the dumbbells slightly greater than shoulder-width apart at the level of your chest with the palms of your hands facing each other and your elbows bent at 90 degrees with upper arms parallel to the floor [1]. In one curved motion, push the dumbbells upward by straightening your arms and bring the dumbbells in toward the midline of your chest while rotating your hands so that your palms face away from you as the ends of the dumbbells meet [2]. Lower the dumbbells back along the same arc to the level of your chest and repeat for the prescribed number of reps.

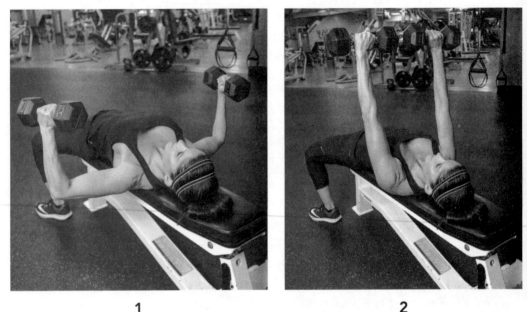

1   2

Dumbbell Lunges

Stand with your torso upright, holding a dumbbell in each hand by your sides [1]. Step forward about two feet with your right leg and lower yourself down into the lunge while keeping your torso upright. Keep your right knee above your toes as you lunge forward and keep your right shin perpendicular to the ground [2]. Push yourself back up and lunge forward with your left leg. Repeat for the prescribed number of reps.

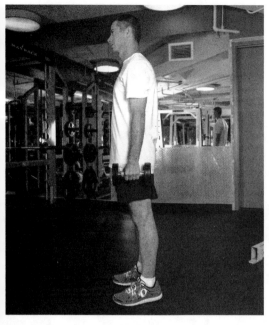

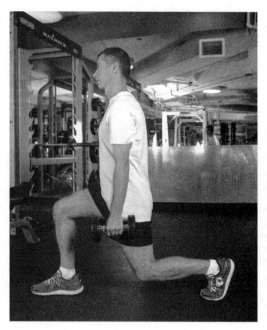

1   2

Dumbbell Reverse Flys

Grab a dumbbell in each hand with an overhand grip and palms facing each other and stand with feet shoulder-width apart. Slightly bend your knees and lean forward from your hips with your back straight. Hold the dumbbells with your arms slightly bent [1]. Raise your arms out to your sides like a fly opening its wings until your elbows are slightly higher than your shoulders [2]. Lower the dumbbells to the starting position and repeat for the prescribed number of reps. You can also do this exercise on an incline bench with your torso flat against the bench [3 & 4].

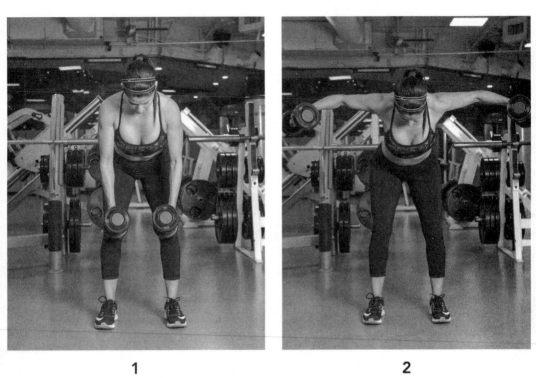

1

2

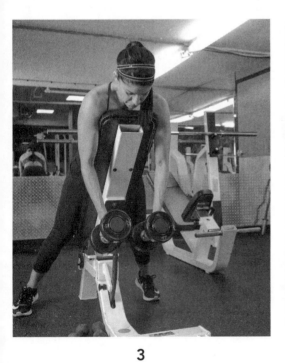

3

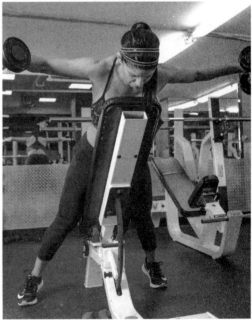

4

14-MINUTE METABOLIC WORKOUTS

Dumbbell Deadlift

Hold a dumbbell in each hand by your sides at arm's length and stand with your feet shoulder-width apart [1]. Keeping your back and legs straight, bend over at the waist to lower the dumbbells until your back is parallel to the floor. As you bend over, you should feel a stretch in your hamstrings [2]. Keeping your back and legs straight, stand upright to return to the starting position and repeat for the prescribed number of reps.

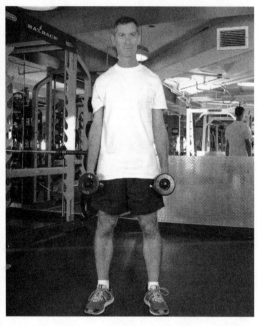

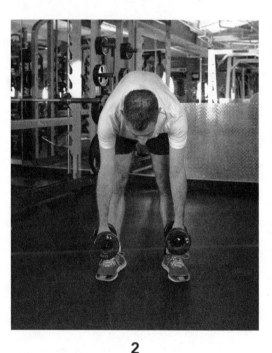

1

2

Dumbbell Row

Stand with feet shoulder-width apart with knees slightly bent and hold a dumbbell in each hand with palms facing each other. Keeping your back straight, bend over at the waist until your back is almost parallel to the floor. The dumbbells should hang directly in front of you as your arms hang perpendicular to the floor and your torso [1]. While keeping your torso stationary, use your shoulder muscles to lift the dumbbells, keeping your elbows close to your body [2]. Slowly lower the dumbbells to the starting position and repeat for the prescribed number of reps.

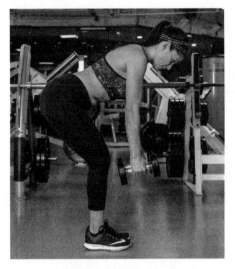
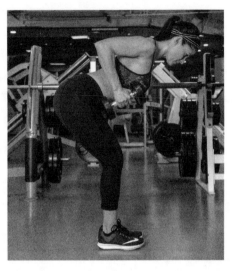

1   2

Dumbbell Calf Raises

Hold a dumbbell in each hand and stand with legs together, with one foot off the ground [1]. With the other foot, push against the ground with the ball of your foot to raise yourself up [2]. Slowly return to the starting position and repeat for the prescribed number of reps.

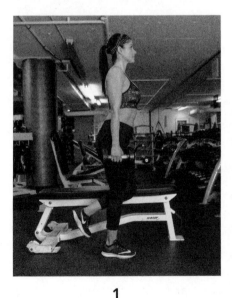
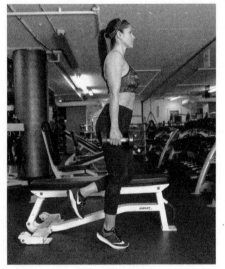

1   2

Dumbbell Biceps Curls

Stand with feet shoulder-width apart and your back straight. Hold a dumbbell in each hand with your arms by your sides. Keep your elbows close to your body [1]. Lift the dumbbells by bending your elbows and rotate your hands so that your palms face up as the dumbbells reach your shoulders [2]. Lower the dumbbells to the starting position and repeat for the prescribed number of reps.

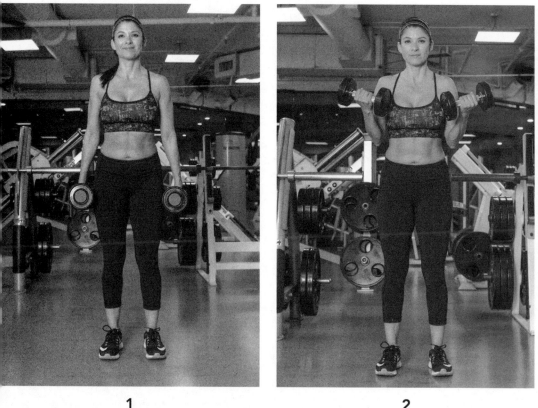

1   2

BODY WEIGHT WORKOUTS

Upper Body 1: Back & Abs

Exercise	Sets	Reps	Recovery
Scissors	3–4	10–20	:30
Superman	3–4	10–20	:30
Pike Crunches	3–4	10–20	:30

EXERCISE INSTRUCTIONS

Scissors

Lie on the ground on your back with your hands at your sides. Squeeze your core so that your shoulders are slightly off the ground. Keeping your legs straight, lift them a few inches off the ground and scissor kick them in the air by moving them up and down [1 & 2]. Repeat the scissor-kick motion for the prescribed number of reps without letting your legs or feet touch the ground.

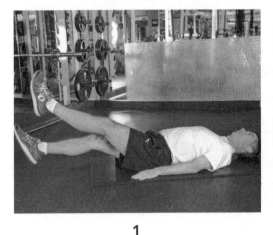

1

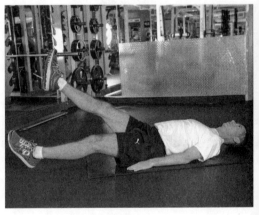

2

Superman

Lie facedown on the ground, legs together and straight, and arms straight and extended above your head. Keep your head and neck in a neutral position [1]. Simultaneously raise your arms, legs, and chest off the floor and hold this position for two seconds. You should look like Superman flying to save Lois Lane [2]. Slowly lower your arms, legs, and chest back down to the starting position and repeat for the prescribed number of reps.

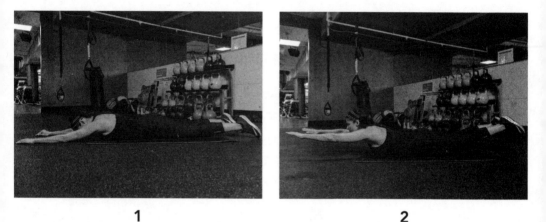

1   2

Pike Crunches

Lie on your back on the ground with your arms outstretched above your head and legs straight out [1]. In one smooth motion, and without straining your neck, lift your torso off the ground while lifting your legs so that your arms and legs meet in the middle in a pike position [2]. Slowly lower your torso and legs back down to the starting position and repeat for the prescribed number of reps. You can modify this exercise by holding a stability ball between your ankles.

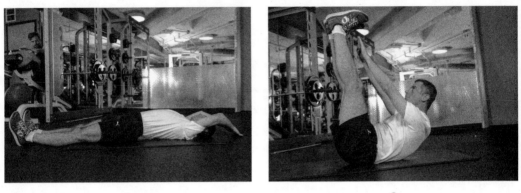

1 2

Upper Body 2: Chest, Shoulders, & Triceps

Exercise	Sets	Reps	Recovery
Push-Ups	3–4	10–20	:30
Shoulder Stabilizers	3–4	10–20	:30
Triceps Dips	3–4	10–20	:30

EXERCISE INSTRUCTIONS

Push-Ups

Assume a standard push-up position, with legs lifted off the ground and back straight. Place your hands together so that your touching forefingers and thumbs form a diamond [1]. Lower yourself down until your chest comes close to the ground [2]. Push yourself back up to the starting position until your arms are straight and repeat for the prescribed number of reps. You can modify this push-up position by placing your knees on the ground and flexed to 90 degrees with ankles crossed [3 & 4], by doing standard push-ups with hands shoulder-width apart, or by placing your hands on a bench [5 & 6].

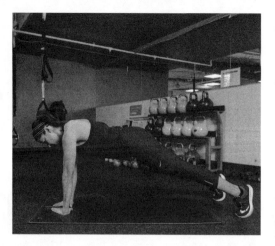

1

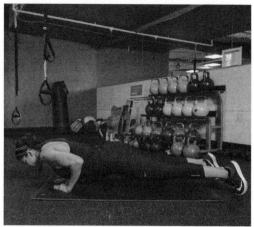

2

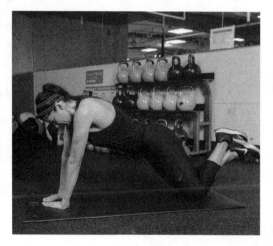

3

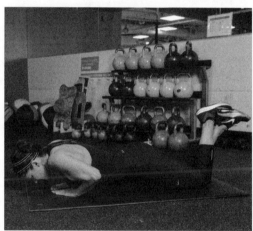

4

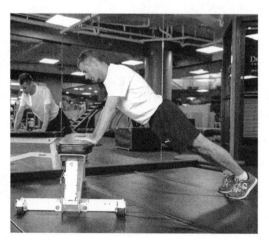

5

6

MUSCULAR ENDURANCE WORKOUTS

Shoulder Stabilizers

Lie on your stomach on a mat with your arms outstretched overhead and your legs outstretched with your toes pointed down [1]. Lift your arms slightly off the floor and reach your arms out to your sides [2] and across your back [3]. Reverse the motion to return to the starting position and repeat for the prescribed number of reps.

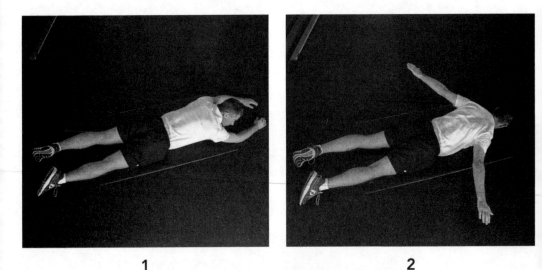

1

2

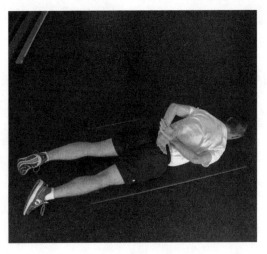

3

Triceps Dips

Stand with your back to a bench, step, or other immovable object. Lower yourself down to the level of the object and hold on to its edge with your arms nearly locked and legs outstretched in front of you. Keep your elbows close to your body [1]. Slowly lower your torso by bending your elbows until your elbow angle is 90 degrees or slightly less [2]. Push your torso back up by using your triceps to bring your body back to the starting position and repeat the movement for the prescribed number of reps. To make the exercise more challenging, place your feet on a bench in front of you rather than on the ground so that your entire body is elevated off the ground.

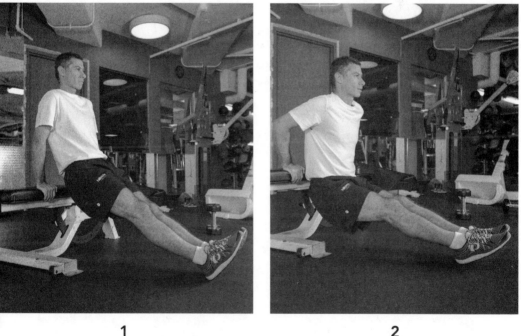

1   2

Lower Body 1: Quads, Glutes, & Calves

Exercise	Sets	Reps	Recovery
Speed Skater	3–4	10–20	:30
Squats with Calf Raise	3–4	10–20	:30
Mountain Climbers	3–4	10–20	:30

EXERCISE INSTRUCTIONS

Speed Skater

Stand with your feet shoulder-width apart. Bend your knees to lower your body into a half squat and lean forward slightly from the waist, sticking your butt out. Shift your weight onto your left leg and pick your right leg up off the floor and place it behind your left ankle [1]. Then, hop sideways to your right by pushing with the outside edge of your left foot and land on your right foot, bringing your left leg behind your right ankle [2]. Swing your arms in concert with your legs so that your right arm is forward when your left leg lands and vice versa. Continue hopping from one side to the other for the prescribed number of reps.

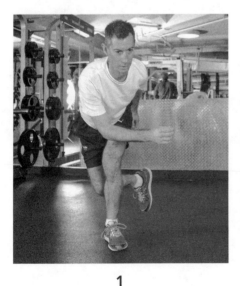
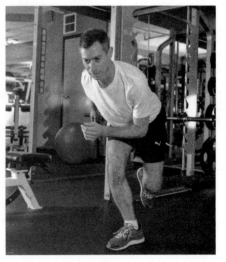

1

2

Squats with Calf Raise

Stand with feet shoulder-width or slightly wider than shoulder-width apart with hands on your hips [1]. Keeping your back straight, bend your knees and squat down until your thighs are parallel to the floor. Move your hips back as if you're going to sit in a chair [2]. Push against the floor to stand up straight and then push with the balls of your feet to raise your heels off the floor as high as they can go so that your weight is almost on your toes [3]. Return to the starting position and repeat for the prescribed number of reps.

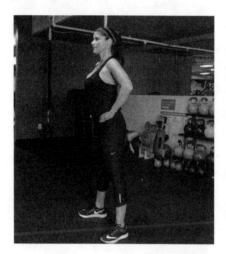

1

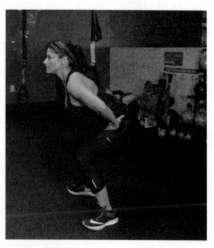

2

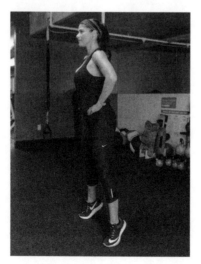

3

Mountain Climbers

Start in a push-up position, with your weight supported by your hands and toes. Bend your right knee and bring your right leg forward until your knee is approximately under your hip [1]. Quickly reverse the position of your legs, extending the bent right leg until it is straight and supported by your toes and bringing your left foot forward with your hip and knee flexed [2]. Repeat by alternating your legs back and forth for the prescribed number of reps.

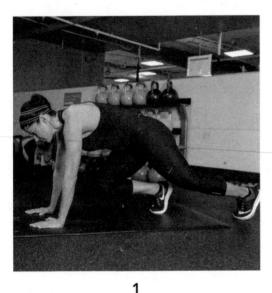

1

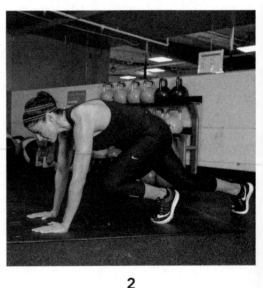

2

Lower Body 2: Hamstrings, Glutes, & Inner Thighs

Exercise	Sets	Reps	Recovery
Squat Side Steps	3–4	10–20	:30
Fencer's Lunge	3–4	10–20	:30
Single-Leg Deadlift	3–4	10–20	:30

EXERCISE INSTRUCTIONS

Squat Side Steps

Stand in a squat position with feet shoulder-width apart and thighs nearly parallel to the floor [1]. Push with your right leg to step laterally to your left while remaining in the squat position [2]. Bring your right foot back to the starting position and continue for the prescribed number of reps before switching to the other direction. Keep your chest up and back straight. To add resistance, use a resistance band or physical therapy band secured around your ankles.

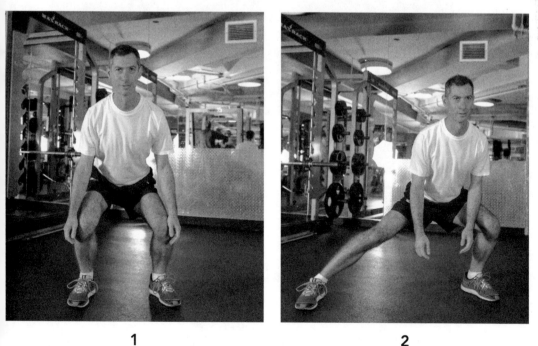

1   2

Fencer's Lunge

Stand with your legs shoulder-width apart. Turn your right leg 90 degrees to your right and turn your body so you are facing to your right. Lunge your right leg forward like a fencer, keeping your back straight, chest out, and shoulders back. Keep your back leg straight. Push off with your right heel to the starting position. Repeat for the prescribed number of reps before switching to your left leg.

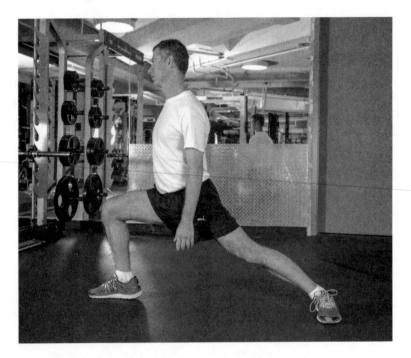

Single-Leg Deadlift

Stand with your feet together [1]. Lift your right leg slightly off the ground and lower your arms and torso while raising your right leg behind you. Keep your left knee slightly bent as you reach forward with your arms as close to the floor as possible [2]. Raise your torso while lowering your right leg to return to the starting position. Repeat for the prescribed number of reps before switching to the other leg.

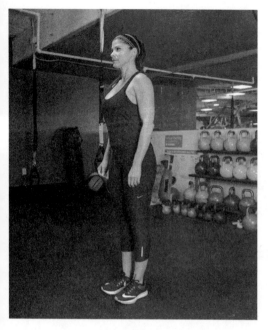

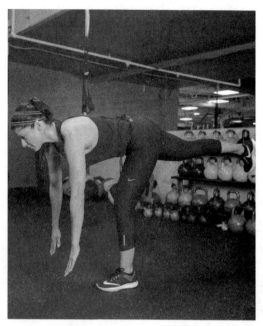

1   2

Total Body Weight Workout

Exercise	Sets	Reps	Recovery
Squats with Calf Raise	1	as many as possible	:30
Push-Ups	1	as many as possible	:30
Single-Leg Deadlift	1	as many as possible	:30
Superman	1	as many as possible	:30
Fencer's Lunge	1	as many as possible	:30
Triceps Dips	1	as many as possible	:30
Mountain Climbers	1	as many as possible	:30
Pike Crunches	1	as many as possible	:30

Exercises alternate between lower body and upper body and progress from bigger muscles to smaller muscles.

Squats with Calf Raise

Stand with feet shoulder-width or slightly wider than shoulder-width apart with hands on your hips [1]. Keeping your back straight, bend your knees and squat down until your thighs are parallel to the floor. Move your hips back as if you're going to sit in a chair [2]. Push against the floor to stand up straight and then push with the balls of your feet to raise your heels off the floor as high as they can go so that your weight is almost on your toes [3]. Return to the starting position and repeat for the prescribed number of reps.

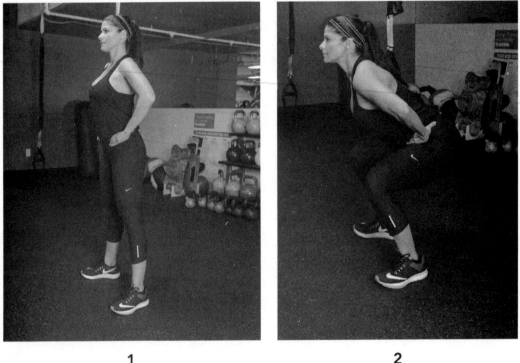

1   2

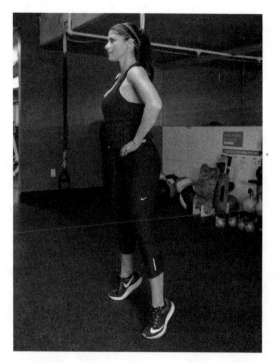

3

Push-Ups

Assume a standard push-up position, with legs lifted off the ground and back straight. Place your hands together so that your touching forefingers and thumbs form a diamond [1]. Lower yourself down until your chest comes close to the ground [2]. Push yourself back up to the starting position until your arms are straight and repeat for the prescribed number of reps. You can modify this push-up position by placing your knees on the ground and flexed to 90 degrees with ankles crossed [3 & 4], by doing standard push-ups with hands shoulder-width apart, or by placing your hands on a bench [5 & 6].

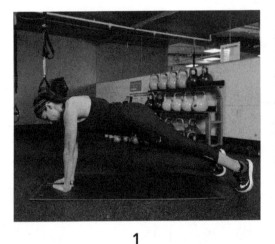

1

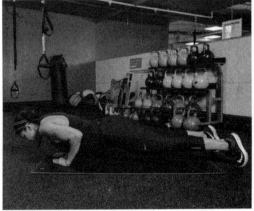

2

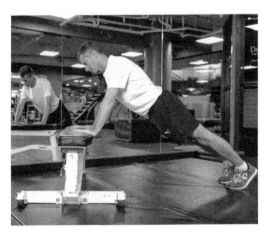

3

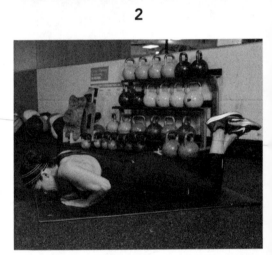

4

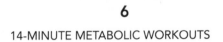

5

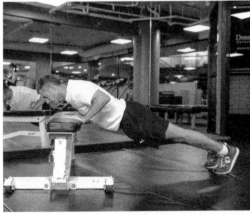

6

14-MINUTE METABOLIC WORKOUTS

Single-Leg Deadlift

Stand with your feet together [1]. Lift your right leg slightly off the ground and lower your arms and torso while raising your right leg behind you. Keep your left knee slightly bent as you reach forward with your arms as close to the floor as possible [2]. Raise your torso while lowering your right leg to return to the starting position. Repeat for the prescribed number of reps before switching to the other leg.

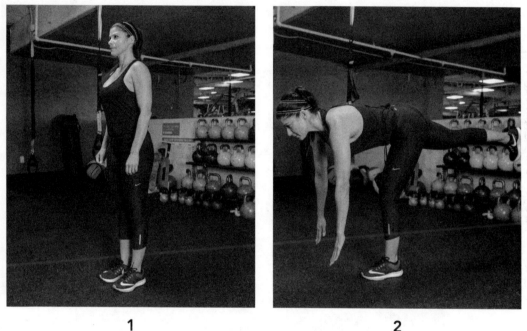

1   2

Superman

Lie facedown on the ground, legs together and straight, and arms straight and extended above your head. Keep your head and neck in a neutral position [1]. Simultaneously raise your arms, legs, and chest off the floor and hold this position for two seconds. You should look like Superman flying to save Lois Lane [2]. Slowly lower your arms, legs, and chest back down to the starting position and repeat for the prescribed number of reps.

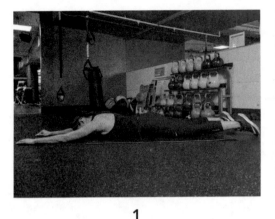

1

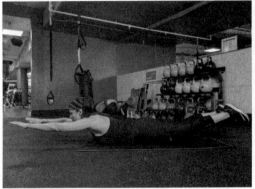

2

Fencer's Lunge

Stand with your legs shoulder-width apart. Turn your right leg 90 degrees to your right and turn your body so you are facing to your right. Lunge your right leg forward like a fencer, keeping your back straight, chest out, and shoulders back. Keep your back leg straight. Push off with your right heel to the starting position. Repeat for the prescribed number of reps before switching to your left leg.

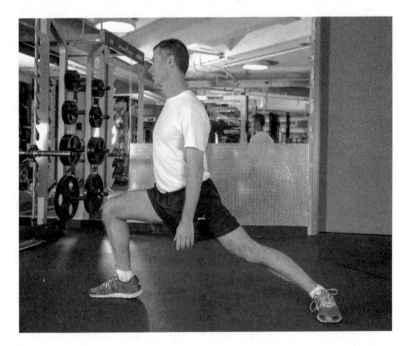

Triceps Dips

Stand with your back to a bench, step, or other immovable object. Lower yourself down to the level of the object and hold on to its edge with your arms nearly locked and legs outstretched in front of you. Keep your elbows close to your body [1]. Slowly lower your torso by bending your elbows until your elbow angle is 90 degrees or slightly less [2]. Push your torso back up by using your triceps to bring your body back to the starting position and repeat the movement for the prescribed number of reps. To make the exercise more challenging, place your feet on a bench in front of you rather than on the ground so that your entire body is elevated off the ground.

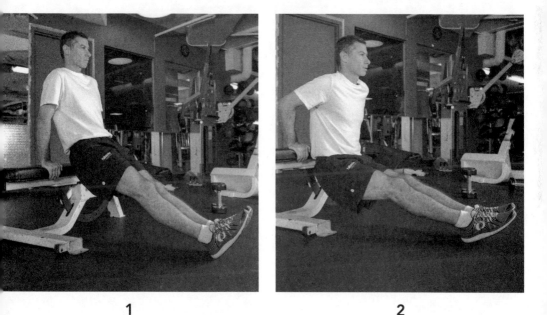

1   2

Mountain Climbers

Start in a push-up position, with your weight supported by your hands and toes. Bend your right knee and bring your right leg forward until your knee is approximately under your hip [1]. Quickly reverse the position of your legs, extending the bent right leg until it is straight and supported by your toes and bringing your left foot forward with your hip and knee flexed

[2]. Repeat by alternating your legs back and forth for the prescribed number of reps.

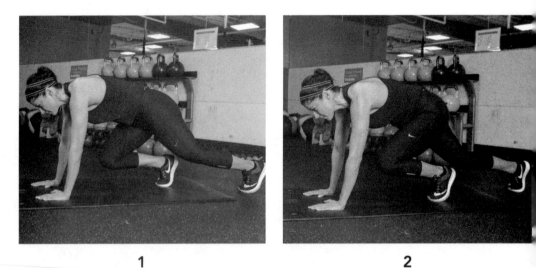

1   2

Pike Crunches

Lie on your back on the ground with your arms outstretched above your head and legs straight out [1]. In one smooth motion, and without straining your neck, lift your torso off the ground while lifting your legs so that your arms and legs meet in the middle in a pike position [2]. Slowly lower your torso and legs back down to the starting position and repeat for the prescribed number of reps. You can modify this exercise by holding a stability ball between your ankles.

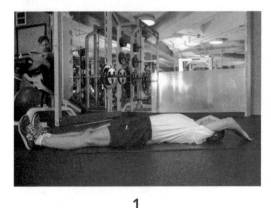
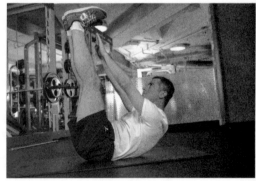

1   2

CIRCUIT WORKOUTS

Dumbbell Total-Body Circuit

Exercise	Reps
Dumbbell Single-Arm Swings	10–20 each arm
Chest Press Sit-Ups	10–20
Dumbbell Discus	10–20 each side
Renegades	10–20 each arm
Squat to Overhead Press	10–20
Dumbbell Russian Twists	10–20 each side

Go immediately from one exercise to the next. Do the circuit once or twice with a 2-minute rest between circuits.

EXERCISE INSTRUCTIONS

Dumbbell Single-Arm Swings

Stand up straight with feet slightly wider than shoulder-width apart. Grab the dumbbell with your right hand, keeping your palm facedown and arm in front of your body. Bend your knees slightly and drive your hips back as you swing the dumbbell between your legs [1]. Explosively drive your hips forward while swinging the dumbbell upward until your arm is parallel to the ground [2]. Swing the dumbbell back down to the starting position and quickly transfer it to your left hand as it passes through your legs. Repeat the swing with your left arm and continue alternating hands for the prescribed number of reps.

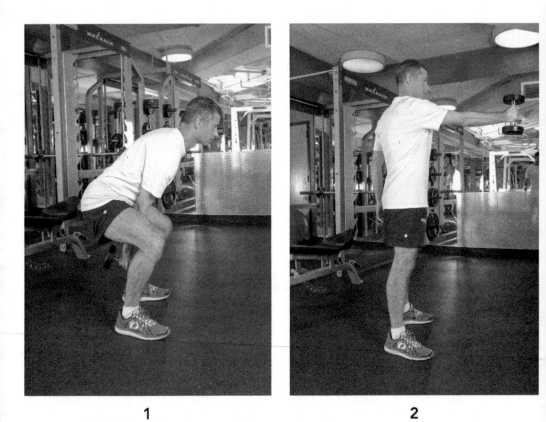

1   2

Chest Press Sit-Ups

Lie on the ground with your legs bent and feet on the floor
and anchored under an immovable object. Hold the dumbbell
at its ends with both hands close to your chest [1]. Push the
dumbbell up away from your chest as you lift your head slightly
off the ground [2]. Lower the dumbbell and raise your torso off
the ground to do a sit-up [3]. Lower your torso back down to
the ground and repeat for the prescribed number of reps.

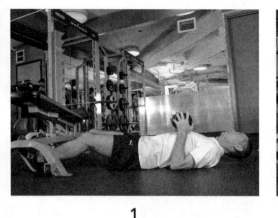

1

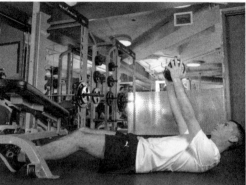

2

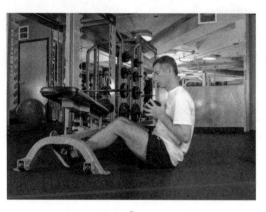

3

Dumbbell Discus

Stand with legs shoulder-width apart, with your left leg slightly in front of your right. Hold the dumbbell in your right hand down at your side. Bend your knees and squat down to about a quarter to a half squat. Pivot with your feet and twist to your right, bringing your left arm across your body to meet your right hand and dumbbell [1]. Pivot your feet and use your hips to quickly twist your body to your left as you stand up out of the squat. As you twist to your left, raise the dumbbell across your chest with your arms extended from your lower right side to your upper left side, meeting the end of the dumbbell to your outstretched left hand [2]. Reverse the movement to return to the starting position and repeat for the prescribed number of reps before switching to the other side.

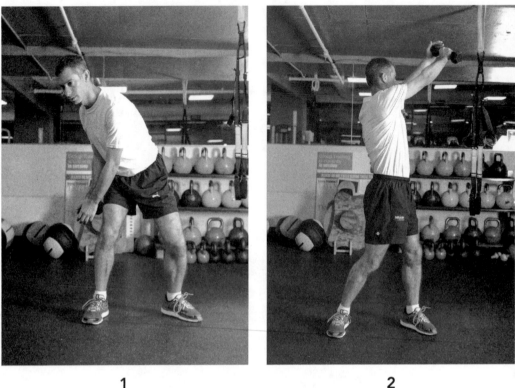

1　　　　　　　　**2**

Renegades

Stand with your legs shoulder-width apart, bend at the waist, and hold a dumbbell in each hand with arms hanging down in front of you and palms facing each other [1]. Bend your right elbow to quickly pull the dumbbell to your chest [2]. Lower that dumbbell and quickly pull the dumbbell in your left hand to your chest [3]. Keep alternating arms and repeat for the prescribed number of reps.

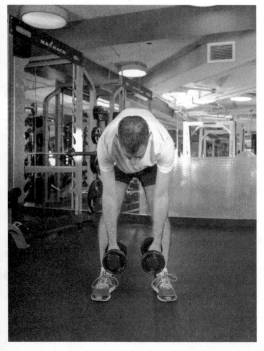

1

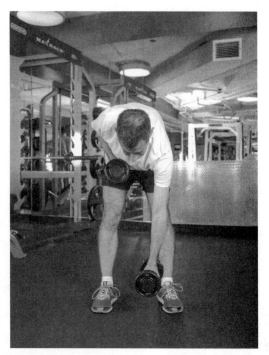

2

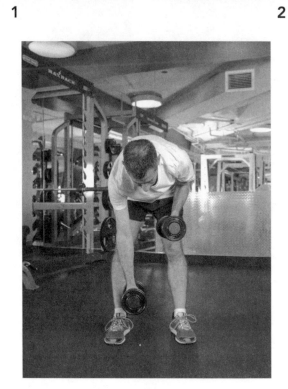

3

Squat to Overhead Press

Stand with feet shoulder-width apart with a dumbbell in each hand near your shoulders with elbows bent at 90 degrees and pointing down and palms facing each other [1]. Keeping your back straight, bend your knees and squat down until your thighs are parallel to the floor. Move your hips back as if you're going to sit in a chair [2]. Push against the floor to stand up and press the dumbbells up until your arms are extended [3]. Lower the dumbbells back to the starting position, keeping the weight balanced over your elbows, and repeat for the prescribed number of reps.

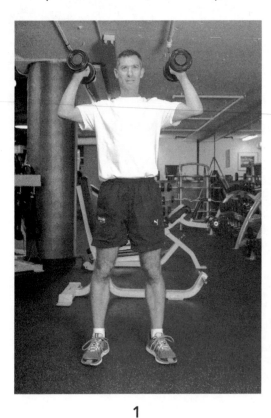

1

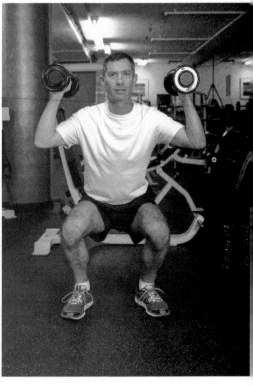

2

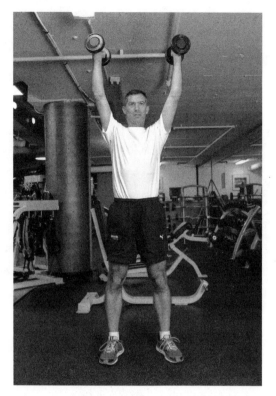

3

Dumbbell Russian Twists

Sit on the ground with your legs bent and feet anchored under an immovable object. Lean your torso back so that your butt creates a V shape with your thighs. Hold the dumbbell at its ends with both hands close to your chest [1]. Twist your torso as far as you can to your left side [2]. Hold this position for a brief moment and then twist your torso to your right side. Continue to twist to your right and left sides for the prescribed number of reps.

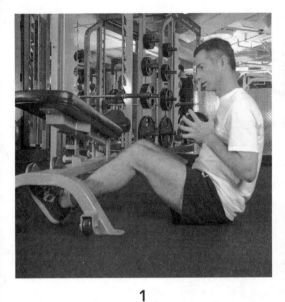
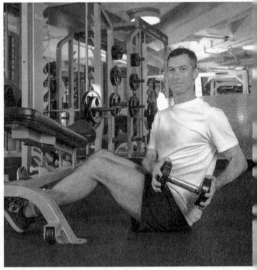

1   2

Sprint/Body Weight Circuit

Exercise	Duration/Reps
Sprint	:30
Squat Jumps	10–15
Push-Ups	10–15
Pike Crunches	10–15
Sprint	:30
Squat Side Steps	10–15 each side
Superman	10–15
V-Sit	10–15
Sprint	:30
Mountain Climbers	10–15 each leg
Triceps Dips	10–15
Russian Twists	10–15

This circuit sequences sprint running with a lower-body exercise, upper-body exercise, and core exercise for a total-body workout. Go immediately from one exercise to the next. Do the circuit once or twice with a 2-minute rest between circuits. If you do this workout in a gym, you can substitute sprint cycling for sprint running. Make the sprint fast and challenging, but not all out.

EXERCISE INSTRUCTIONS

Squat Jumps

Begin in a squat position with thighs parallel to the ground and hands on your hips [1]. Jump straight up as high as you can [2]. Land with soft knees, lowering yourself back into the squat position in one smooth motion, and immediately jump up again. Repeat for the prescribed number of reps.

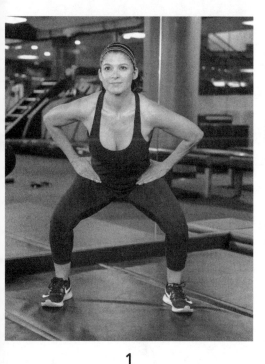

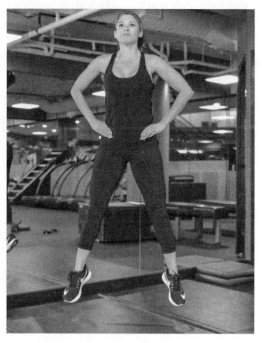

1   2

Push-Ups

Assume a standard push-up position, with legs lifted off the ground and back straight. Place your hands together so that your touching forefingers and thumbs form a diamond [1]. Lower yourself down until your chest comes close to the ground [2]. Push yourself back up to the starting position until your arms are straight and repeat for the prescribed number of reps. You can modify this push-up position by placing your knees on the ground and flexed to 90 degrees with ankles crossed [3 & 4], by doing standard push-ups with hands shoulder-width apart, or by placing your hands on a bench [5 & 6].

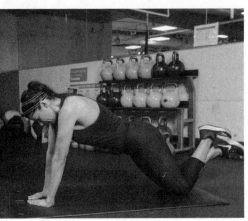

1

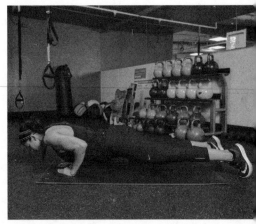

2

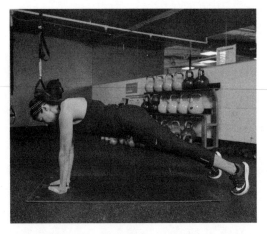

3

4

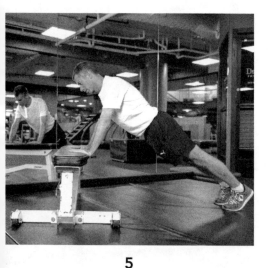

5

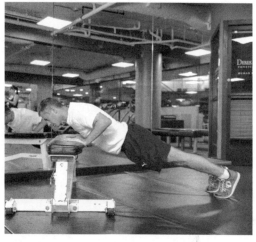

6

Pike Crunches

Lie on your back on the ground with your arms outstretched above your head and legs straight out [1]. In one smooth motion, and without straining your neck, lift your torso off the ground while lifting your legs so that your arms and legs meet in the middle in a pike position [2]. Slowly lower your torso and legs back down to the starting position and repeat for the prescribed number of reps. You can modify this exercise by holding a stability ball between your ankles.

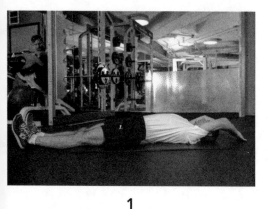

1

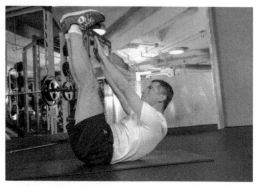

2

Squat Side Steps

Stand in a squat position with feet shoulder-width apart and thighs nearly parallel to the floor [1]. Push with your right leg to step laterally to your left while remaining in the squat position [2]. Bring your right foot back to the starting position and continue for the prescribed number of reps before switching to the other direction. Keep your chest up and back straight. To add resistance, use a resistance band or physical therapy band secured around your ankles.

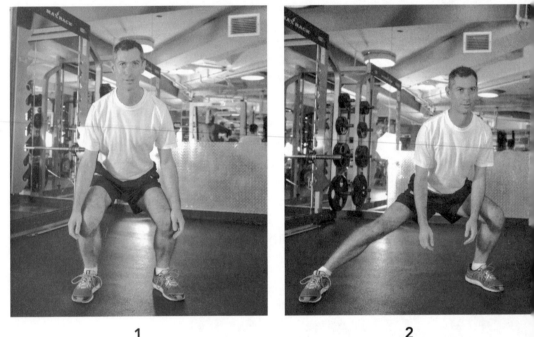

1   2

Superman

Lie facedown on the ground, legs together and straight, and arms straight and extended above your head. Keep your head and neck in a neutral position [1]. Simultaneously raise your arms, legs, and chest off the floor and hold this position for two seconds. You should look like Superman flying to save Lois Lane [2]. Slowly lower your arms, legs, and chest back down to the starting position and repeat for the prescribed number of reps.

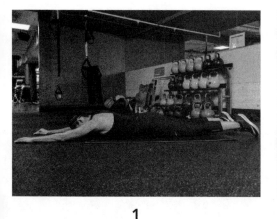

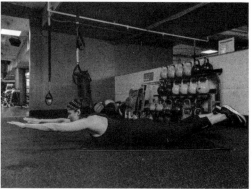

| 1 | 2 |

V-Sit

Sit on the ground in a laid-back position, with your legs raised off the ground. Lean back and place your hands on the ground near your hips for support [1]. Contract your abs to lift your torso while simultaneously bringing your knees toward your chest to create a V shape (your hips should be the point of the V as you balance on your buttocks in the V position) [2]. Repeat for the prescribed number of reps.

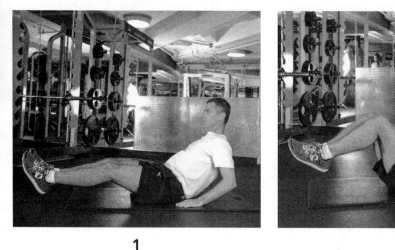

| 1 | 2 |

Mountain Climbers

Start in a push-up position, with your weight supported by your hands and toes. Bend your right knee and bring your right leg forward until your knee is approximately under your hip [1]. Quickly reverse the position of your legs, extending the bent right leg until it is straight and supported by your toes and bringing your left foot forward with your hip and knee flexed [2]. Repeat by alternating your legs back and forth for the prescribed number of reps.

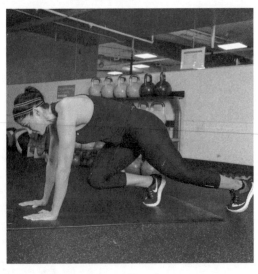

1

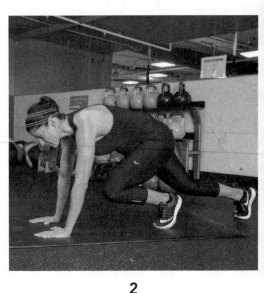

2

Triceps Dips

Stand with your back to a bench, step, or other immovable object. Lower yourself down to the level of the object and hold on to its edge with your arms nearly locked and legs outstretched in front of you. Keep your elbows close to your body [1]. Slowly lower your torso by bending your elbows until your elbow angle is 90 degrees or slightly less [2]. Push your torso back up by using your triceps to bring your body back to the starting position and repeat the movement for the prescribed number of reps. To make the exercise more challenging, place your feet on a bench in front of you rather than on the ground so that your entire body is elevated off the ground.

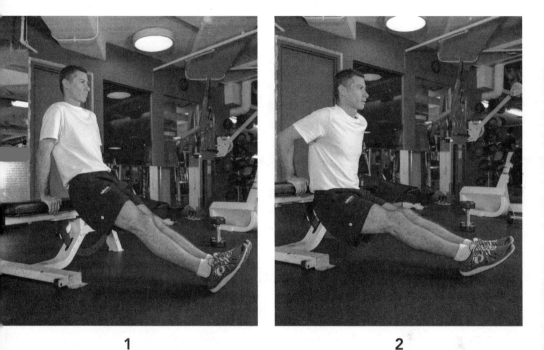

1   **2**

Russian Twists

Sit on the ground with your legs bent and feet anchored under an immovable object. Lean your torso back so that your butt creates a V shape with your thighs. Hold your arms extended in front of you with your hands clasped [1]. Twist your torso as far as you can to your right side [2]. Hold this position for a brief moment and then twist your torso to your left side. Continue to twist to your right and left sides for the prescribed number of reps. To make the exercise more challenging, hold a dumbbell or other weighted object in your hands as you twist from side to side.

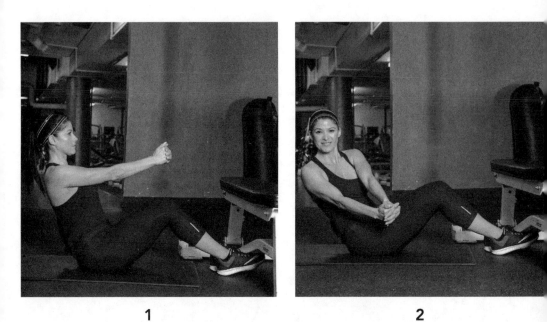

1   2

Core Circuit

Exercise	Reps
Russian Twists	10–20 each side
Glute Bridge	10–20
Superman	10–20
Pike Crunches	10–20
Scissors	10–20 each leg
V-Sit	10–20

Go immediately from one exercise to the next and do circuit 2 to 3 times, with a 1-minute rest between circuits.

EXERCISE INSTRUCTIONS

Russian Twists

Sit on the ground with your legs bent and feet anchored under an immovable object. Lean your torso back so that your butt creates a V shape with your thighs. Hold your arms extended in front of you with your hands clasped [1]. Twist your torso as far as you can to your right side [2]. Hold this position for a brief moment and then twist your torso to your left side. Continue to twist to your right and left sides for the prescribed number of reps. To make the exercise more challenging, hold a dumbbell or other weighted object in your hands as you twist from side to side.

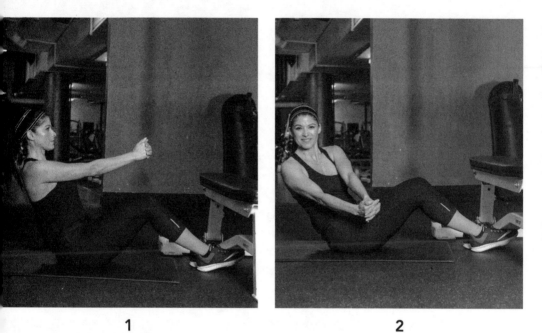

1   2

Glute Bridge

Lie on your back with your knees bent at about 90 degrees and your feet flat on the ground [1]. Pushing from your heels, lift your hips off the ground. Your weight should be supported by your upper back and the heels of your feet [2]. Slowly lower back down to return to the starting position and repeat for the prescribed number of reps. To make the exercise more challenging, lay a weight over your legs near your hips.

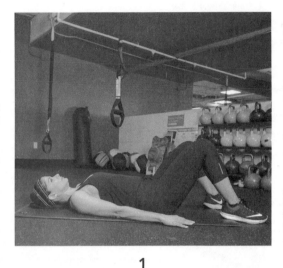

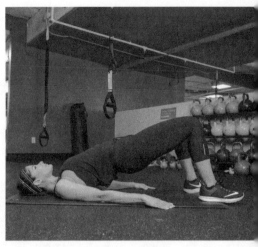

1   2

Superman

Lie facedown on the ground, legs together and straight, and arms straight and extended above your head. Keep your head and neck in a neutral position [1]. Simultaneously raise your arms, legs, and chest off the floor and hold this position for two seconds. You should look like Superman flying to save Lois Lane [2]. Slowly lower your arms, legs, and chest back down to the starting position and repeat for the prescribed number of reps.

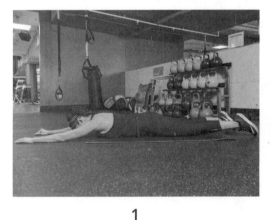

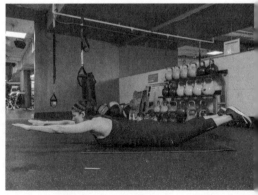

1   2

Pike Crunches

Lie on your back on the ground with your arms outstretched above your head and legs straight out [1]. In one smooth motion, and without straining your neck, lift your torso off the ground while lifting your legs so that your arms and legs meet in the middle in a pike position [2]. Slowly lower your torso and legs back down to the starting position and repeat for the prescribed number of reps. You can modify this exercise by holding a stability ball between your ankles.

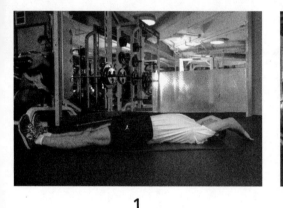

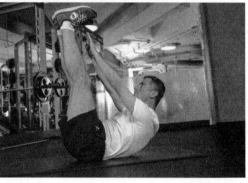

1   2

Scissors

Lie on the ground on your back with your hands at your sides. Squeeze your core so that your shoulders are slightly off the ground. Keeping your legs straight, lift them a few inches off the ground and scissor kick them in the air by moving them up and down [1 & 2]. Repeat the scissor-kick motion for the prescribed number of reps without letting your legs or feet touch the ground.

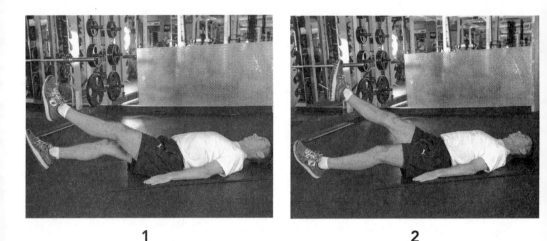

1

2

V-Sit

Sit on the ground in a laid-back position, with your legs raised off the ground. Lean back and place your hands on the ground near your hips for support [1]. Contract your abs to lift your torso while simultaneously bringing your knees toward your chest to create a V shape (your hips should be the point of the V as you balance on your buttocks in the V position) [2]. Repeat for the prescribed number of reps.

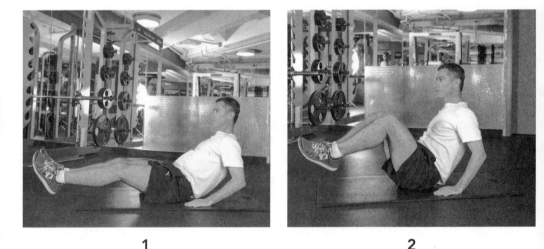

1

2

Resistance Band Circuit

Exercise	Reps
Resistance Band Overhead Press	10–15 each arm
Resistance Band Squat	10–15
Resistance Band Chest Press	10–15
Resistance Band Inner Thigh Pull	10–15 each leg
Resistance Band Bent-Over Row	10–15
Resistance Band Leg Curl	10–15 each leg
Resistance Band Cross-Overs	10–15 each arm
Resistance Band Squat Side Steps	10–15 each leg
Resistance Band Triceps Kickback	10–15
Resistance Band Biceps Curls	10–15

This circuit alternates upper body and lower body exercises, moving from large muscles to small muscles. Go immediately from one exercise to the next.

EXERCISE INSTRUCTIONS

Resistance Band Overhead Press

Stand with feet shoulder-width apart. Hold the handles of the resistance band with elbows bent at 90 degrees and pointing down and palms facing forward [1]. Press the handles up and in together over your head until they meet [2]. Lower the handles back along the same arc to the starting position and repeat for the prescribed number of reps.

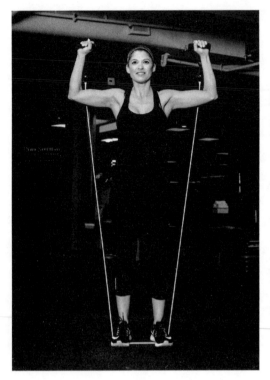
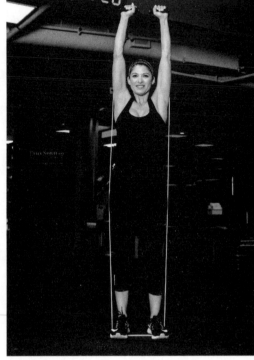

1   2

Resistance Band Squat

Grab both handles of the resistance band with an overhand grip and stand with feet shoulder-width apart on the middle of the band. Make sure equal lengths of the band are on both sides of your body so that they are the same height on each side. Hold the band so it is behind your shoulders with your hands near your shoulders, your elbows pointed down, and your palms facing away from you [1]. Bend your knees as you squat down until your thighs are parallel to the ground [2]. Push through the heels of your feet to stand back up to the starting position and repeat for the prescribed number of reps.

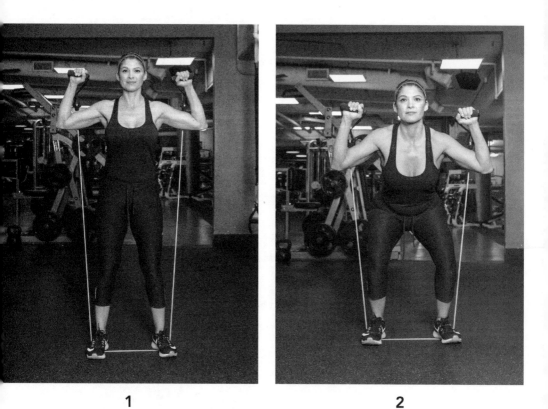

1   2

Resistance Band Chest Press

Wrap the resistance band at chest height around an immovable object. Stand with your back to the object to which you have anchored the band and grab each handle. Step forward a few steps to create enough resistance and stand with one foot slightly in front of the other for balance. Hold the band at chest height with your elbows up and palms facing down [1]. Push the band straight out in front of you until your arms are fully extended [2]. Slowly return to starting position and repeat for the prescribed number of reps.

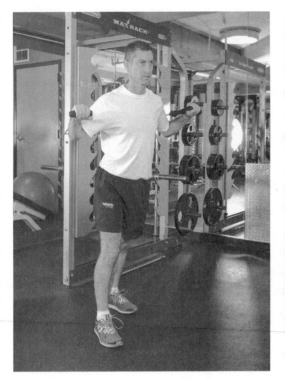
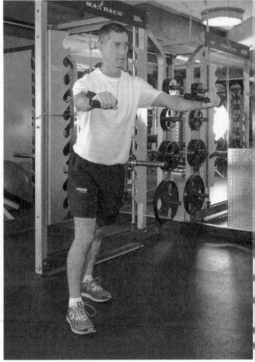

1   2

Resistance Band Inner Thigh Pull

Anchor the resistance band at ankle height to an immovable object and stand with your right side facing the object. Wrap the free end of the band around your right ankle. Stand perpendicular to the band and step away from the object to which the band is anchored to create enough resistance [1]. Lift your right leg slightly off the ground and sweep your right ankle across your body past your left leg [2]. You can lean on a wall for support. Slowly return to the starting position and repeat for the prescribed number of reps before switching to the left leg.

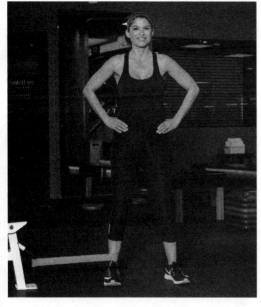
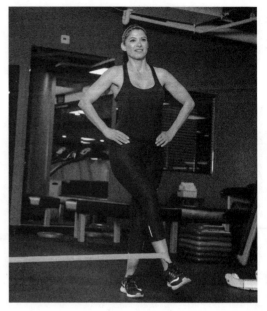

1   2

Resistance Band Bent-Over Row

Stand with your feet shoulder-width apart on the center of the resistance band. Bend your knees slightly and bend over at the waist, keeping your back straight. Hold the handles at shoulder-width with your hands facing each other and arms extended [1]. Pull the band up toward your chest, squeezing your shoulder blades together until your elbows form a 90-degree angle [2]. Slowly return to the starting position and repeat for the prescribed number of reps.

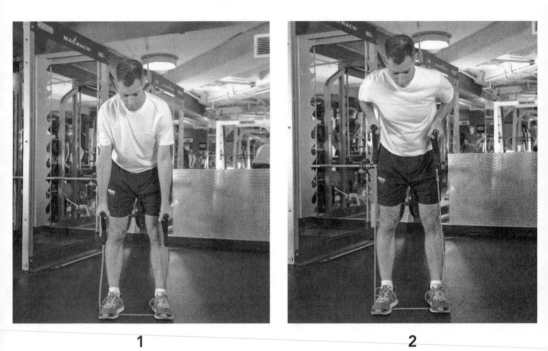

1

2

Resistance Band Leg Curl

Lie facedown and loop the resistance band around your right ankle, anchoring the other end to an immovable object behind you. Move forward from the anchor point to create enough resistance [1]. Bend your knee, curling your right leg up until your heel comes close to your butt [2]. Slowly return to the starting position and repeat for the prescribed number of reps before switching to the left leg.

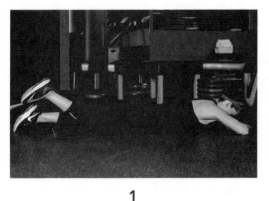

1

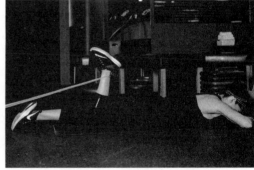

2

Resistance Band Cross-Overs

Stand on the resistance band with your left foot and hold one end of the band with your left hand at the side of your left leg. Hold the other end in your right hand with your right arm across your body so that your right hand meets your left hip [1]. Keeping your arm straight, use your shoulder and upper back muscles to lift your arm up and away from your body until your arm is fully extended [2]. Lower your extended arm back down across your body to return to the starting position and repeat for the prescribed number of reps before switching to the left arm.

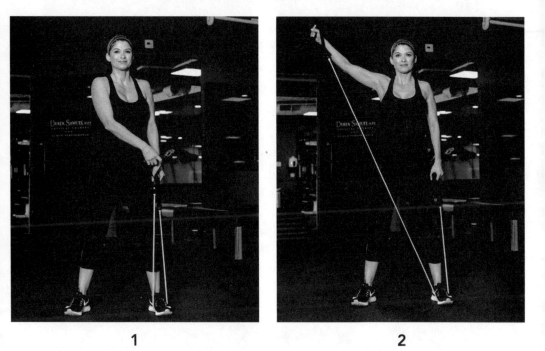

1   2

Resistance Band Squat Side Steps

Secure a resistance band or physical therapy band around your ankles and stand in a squat position with feet shoulder-width apart and thighs nearly parallel to the floor [1]. Push with your right leg to step laterally to your left while remaining in the squat position [2]. Keep your chest up and back straight. Bring your right foot back to the starting position and continue for the prescribed number of reps before switching to the other direction.

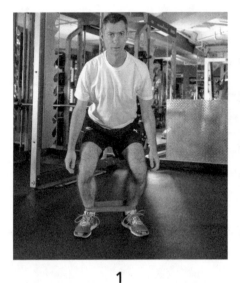

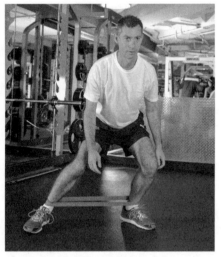

1   2

Resistance Band Triceps Kickback

Stand with your right foot forward in the middle of the resistance band and bend forward at the waist. Grab the handles and hold your arms at your sides with palms facing each other. Keep your arms tucked by your sides with your elbows bent at 90 degrees [1]. Extend your arms back at the elbows until your arms are straight. Only your forearms should move [2]. Return to the starting position and repeat for the prescribed number of reps.

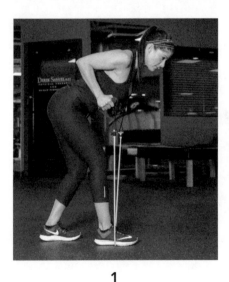

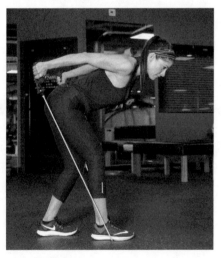

1   2

Resistance Band Biceps Curls

Stand with feet shoulder-width apart and your back straight. Hold the handles of the resistance band with your arms by your sides. Keep your elbows close to your body [1]. Lift the handles by bending your elbows and rotate your hands so that your palms face up as the handles reach your shoulders [2]. Lower the handles to the starting position and repeat for the prescribed number of reps.

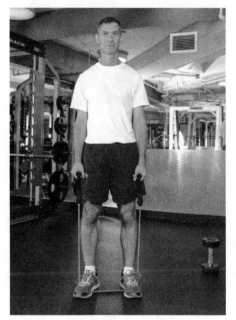

1

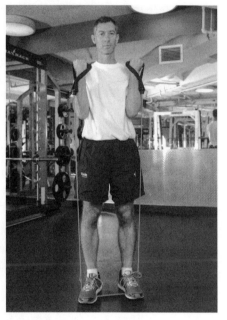

2

Kettlebell Circuit

Exercise	Reps
Kettlebell Swings	10 each arm
Kettlebell Push-Ups with Row	10
Kettlebell Deadlift	10
Kettlebell Russian Twist	10 each side
Kettlebell Goblet Squat	10
Kettlebell Row	10
Kettlebell Squat to Military Press	10

Go immediately from one exercise to the next. Do the circuit once or twice with a 1-minute rest between circuits.

Kettlebell Swings

Stand with feet slightly wider than shoulder-width apart. Grab the handle of the kettlebell with your right hand and arm in front of your body. Bend your knees and drive your hips back as you swing the kettlebell between your legs [1]. Explosively drive your hips forward while swinging the kettlebell upward until your arm is parallel to the ground [2]. Swing the kettlebell back down to the starting position and quickly transfer it to your left hand as it passes through your legs. Repeat the swing with your left arm and continue alternating hands for the prescribed number of reps. You can modify this exercise by holding the kettlebell with both hands [3].

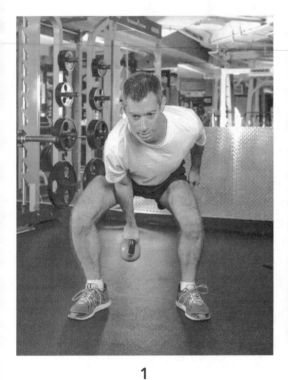

1

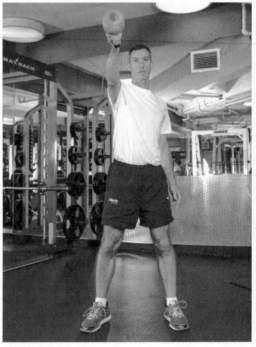

2

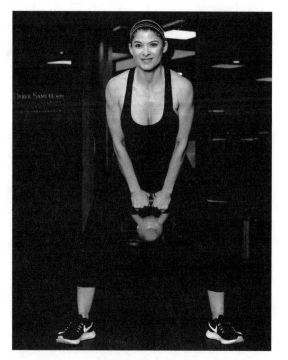

3

Kettlebell Push-Ups with Row

Kneel on the ground, grabbing the handle of a kettlebell in each hand, and place the kettlebells shoulder-width apart. Assume a standard push-up position with your legs off the ground so that just your toes are touching the ground. Keep your back straight [1]. Bend your arms to lower yourself down until your chest meets the level of your hands [2]. Push yourself back up until your arms are straight and add an upright row after completing each push-up by using your shoulder muscles to lift the right kettlebell a few inches off the floor [3]. Lower the kettlebell back to the floor, do another push-up, and do an upright row with your left arm. Repeat for the prescribed number of reps. You can modify this standard push-up position by placing your knees on the ground, flexed to 90 degrees with your ankles crossed.

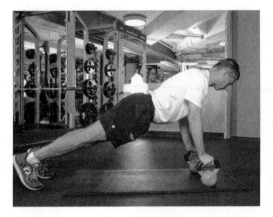

1

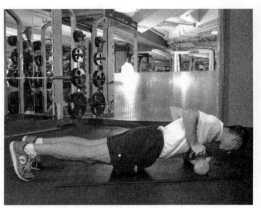

2

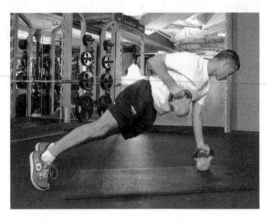

3

Kettlebell Deadlift

Stand with feet slightly greater than shoulder-width apart and the kettlebell between your feet. Keeping your back straight, bend into a quarter squat and grab the handle of the kettlebell with both hands [1]. Stand up, keeping your legs straight [2]. Lower the kettlebell to return to the starting position and repeat for the prescribed number of reps.

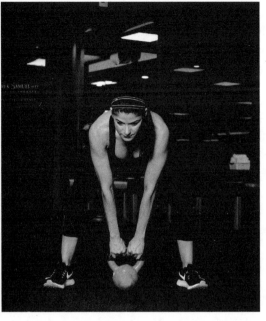
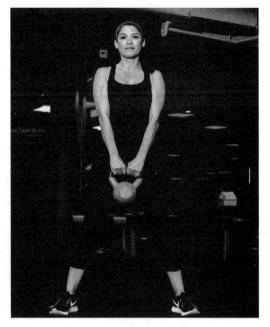

1   2

Kettlebell Russian Twist

Sit on the floor in a laid-back position, leaning back with your torso and knees bent and feet flat on the floor or hanging in the air. Hold the kettlebell with both hands in front of your chest [1]. Twist your torso as far as you can to your left side [2]. Hold this position for a brief moment and then twist your torso to your right side. Continue to twist to your left and right sides for the prescribed number of reps.

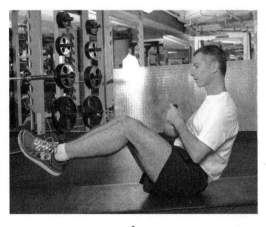

1   2

Kettlebell Goblet Squat

Stand with feet wider than shoulder-width apart and hold the kettlebell with both hands in front of your chest, keeping your elbows close to your body [1]. Keeping your back straight, bend your knees and squat down until your thighs are parallel or lower than parallel to the floor. Move your hips back as if you're going to sit in a chair [2]. Stand up to return to the starting position and repeat for the prescribed number of reps.

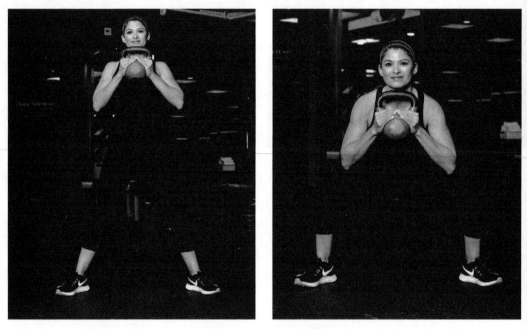

1   2

Kettlebell Row

Grab two kettlebells and stand with feet shoulder-width apart with knees slightly bent. Bend over at the waist [1]. Pull the kettlebells toward your stomach, keeping your back straight and elbows close to your body [2]. Lower the weights to return to the starting position and repeat for the prescribed number of reps.

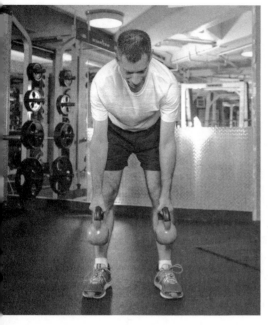

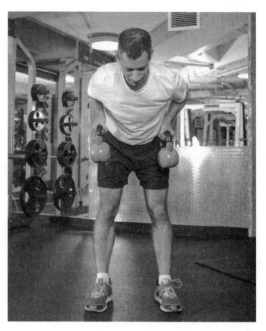

1   2

Kettlebell Squat to Military Press

Stand with feet shoulder-width or slightly wider than shoulder-width apart with a kettlebell in each hand and arms fully extended down at your sides with palms facing the side of your legs [1]. Keeping your back straight, bend your knees and squat down until your thighs are parallel to the ground (the kettlebells will be close to touching the ground) [2]. Push against the ground to return to the starting position as you lift the kettlebells to shoulder height with elbows pointing down [3]. As you reach the standing position, push the kettlebells upward until your arms are fully extended above your head [4]. Slowly return to the starting position and repeat for the prescribed number of reps.

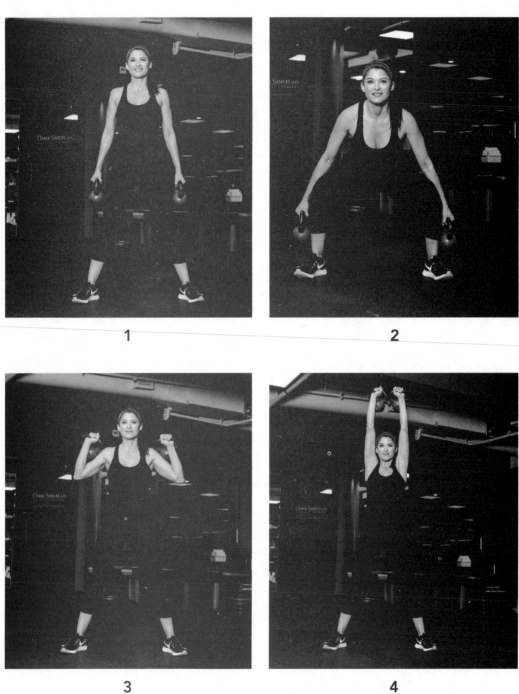

1

2

3

4

14-MINUTE METABOLIC WORKOUTS

TRX Circuit

Exercise	Reps
Single-Leg Squat	10 each leg
Chest Press	10
Hamstring Pull	10
Push-Ups	10
Sprinter's Start	10 each leg
Squat & Row	10
Glute Bridge	10
Biceps Curl	10
Reverse Mountain Climber	10 each leg
Low Row	10

This circuit alternates lower body and upper body suspension exercises using the TRX. Go immediately from one exercise to the next. Do the circuit once or twice with a 1-minute rest between circuits.

EXERCISE INSTRUCTIONS

TRX Single-Leg Squat

Hold both handles of the TRX in front of your chest, with your elbows bent by your sides. Lift your left leg out in front of you [1]. Lower down into a squat on your right leg, extending your arms in front of you at eye level [2]. Push yourself back up to the starting position and repeat for the prescribed number of reps before switching to the left leg.

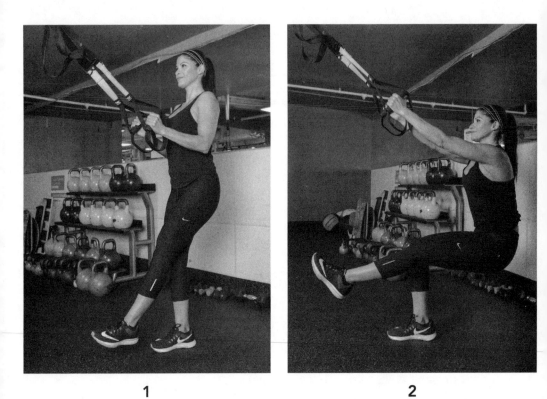

1   2

TRX Chest Press

Stand with your back to the TRX with your feet shoulder-width apart. Grab the handles with an overhand grip and extend your arms in front of you at shoulder height. Lean forward slightly so that your weight is over the balls of your feet [1]. Bend your elbows and lower your chest between your hands [2]. Push yourself back to the starting position and repeat for the prescribed number of reps.

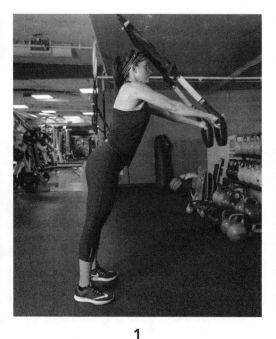
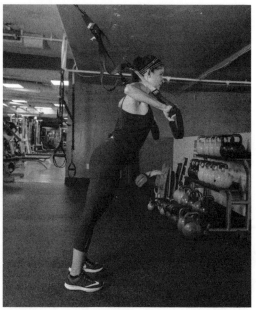

1 **2**

TRX Hamstring Pull

Lie on your back with your legs straight out in front of you and your arms extended by your sides. Secure your feet in the cradles [1]. Lift your hips off the floor and pull your heels in toward your hips [2]. Straighten your legs back to the starting position and repeat for the prescribed number of reps.

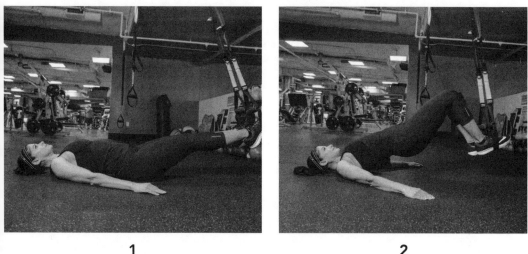

1 **2**

TRX Push-Ups

Assume a push-up position with your feet hooked through the TRX straps. Lift your body up so that your body weight is on your hands [1]. Keeping your core tight, bend your elbows to lower your chest to the floor [2]. Press back up to the starting position and repeat for the prescribed number of reps.

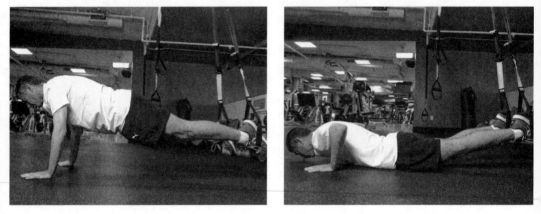

1   2

TRX Sprinter's Start

Stand with your back to the TRX and grab the handles in front of your chest. Lean forward, shifting your weight to the balls of your feet until the straps become taut [1]. Keep your core engaged and drive your right knee forward until your right thigh is parallel to the floor [2]. Pause at the top of the movement, return to the starting position, and repeat for the prescribed number of reps before switching to the left leg.

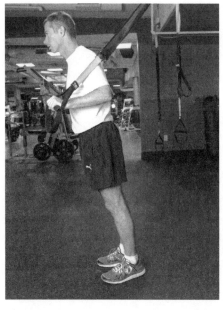

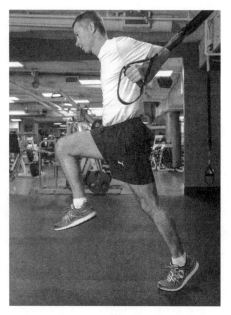

1   2

TRX Squat & Row

Stand facing the TRX and grab the handles with outstretched arms. Step forward and lean back until your arms are in line with your shoulders [1]. Lower down into a squat, using the TRX straps to help you keep your balance [2]. Stand back up and pull on the TRX to bring your chest to your hands [3]. Repeat for the prescribed number of reps.

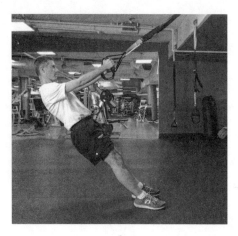

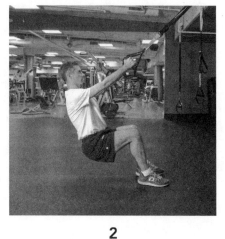

1   2

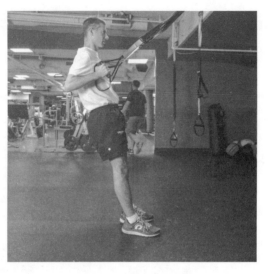

3

TRX Glute Bridge

Lie on your back with your arms extended out to your sides and secure your feet in the cradles. Bring your heels close to your hips until your knees form a 90-degree angle [1]. Lift your butt until your hips are in line with your thighs and torso [2]. Lower your butt back down to the starting position and repeat for the prescribed number of reps.

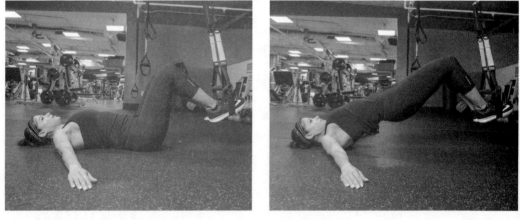

1   **2**

TRX Biceps Curl

Face the TRX and grab the handles with palms facing up. Lean back until your arms are extended and the strap is taut [1]. Pull your body up by keeping your elbows in the same location and bending your elbows until your hands reach the sides of your head [2]. Lower your body back down to return to the starting position and repeat for the prescribed number of reps.

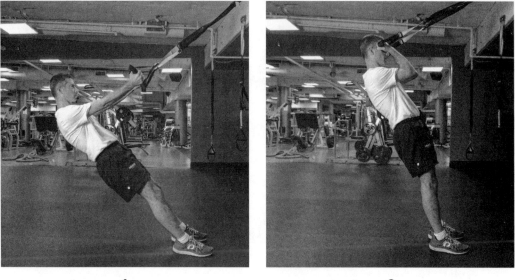

1   2

TRX Reverse Mountain Climber

Sit underneath the TRX and hook your heels into the foot cradles. Place your palms on the floor behind you with your fingers pointed toward your feet. Lift your body off the ground, keeping your elbows slightly bent [1]. Bring your right knee into your chest [2]. Extend your right leg back to the start and immediately bring your left knee into your chest. Repeat for the prescribed number of reps.

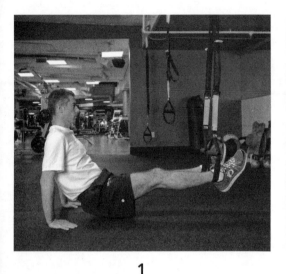

1

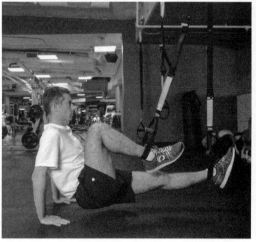

2

TRX Low Row

Grab the handles with your palms facing each other. Lean back until your weight is on your heels and your arms are fully extended in front of you [1]. Squeeze your shoulder blades together and keep your core tight as you bend your elbows and pull your torso up to meet your hands [2]. Lower yourself back down to return to the starting position and repeat for the prescribed number of reps.

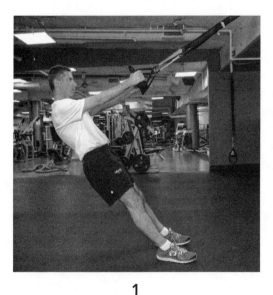

1

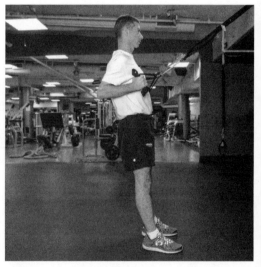

2

Short Circuit 1

Exercise	Reps
High Knees	15–25 each leg
Push-Ups with Dumbbell Row	10–15
V-Sit	15–25

Go immediately from one exercise to the next and do circuit 3 to 5 times, with no rest between circuits.

EXERCISE INSTRUCTIONS

High Knees

Stand with legs shoulder-width apart. Push from the balls of your feet to move your legs up and down quickly as if you're running in place, raising your knees until your thighs are parallel to the ground. Keep your lower leg perpendicular to your thigh so that your knee is at 90 degrees. Lower each leg so that it lands on the ground directly underneath your hips. Think of the ground as hot coals, picking each leg up as soon as it touches the ground. Continue for the prescribed number of reps with each leg.

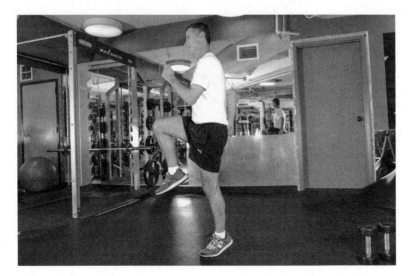

Push-Ups with Dumbbell Row

Kneel on the ground, grabbing an octagon-shaped dumbbell in each hand, and place the dumbbells vertically on the ground shoulder-width apart so that your palms are facing each other. Assume a standard push-up position with your back straight and your legs off the ground so that only your toes are touching the ground [1]. Bend your arms to lower yourself down until your chest comes close to your hands [2]. Push yourself back up until your arms are straight and add an upright row after completing the push-up by using your shoulder muscles to lift the right dumbbell a few inches off the ground [3]. Lower the dumbbell back to the ground, do another push-up, and do an upright row with your left arm. Repeat for the prescribed number of reps. You can modify this standard push-up position by placing your knees on the ground, flexed to 90 degrees with your ankles crossed [4–6].

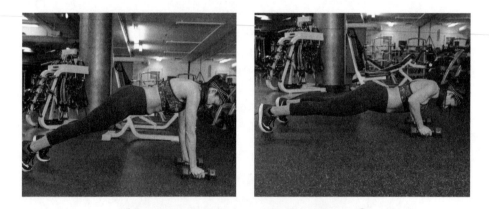

1   2

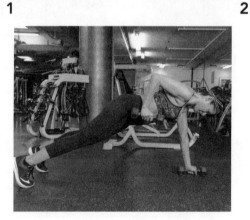

3

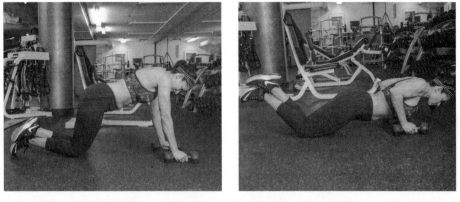

4   5

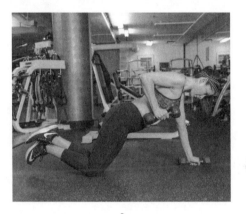

6

V-Sit

Sit on the ground in a laid-back position, with your legs raised off the ground. Lean back and place your hands on the ground near your hips for support [1]. Contract your abs to lift your torso while simultaneously bringing your knees toward your chest to create a V shape (your hips should be the point of the V as you balance on your buttocks in the V position) [2]. Repeat for the prescribed number of reps.

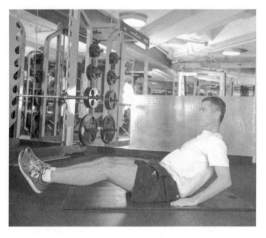

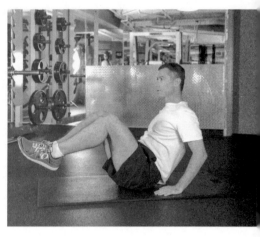

1   2

Short Circuit 2

Exercise	Reps
Split-Jump Lunges	15–25
Overhead Press	15–25
Stair Hops	15–25 each leg

Go immediately from one exercise to the next and do circuit 3 to 5 times, with no rest between circuits.

EXERCISE INSTRUCTIONS

Split-Jump Lunges

Stand with your feet shoulder-width apart. Step forward about two feet with your right leg and lower yourself down into the lunge while keeping your torso upright. Keep your right knee above your toes as you lunge forward and keep your right shin perpendicular to the ground [1]. From this lunge position, jump up into the air with both feet while switching your leg position in midair [2] and land with your left leg forward [3]. Repeat for the prescribed number of reps.

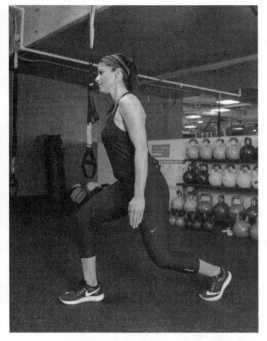

1

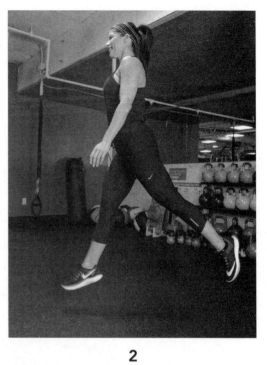

2

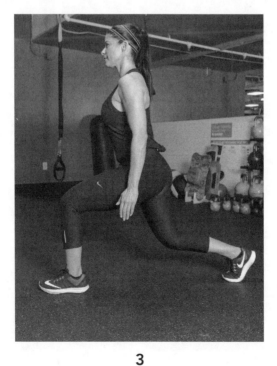

3

Overhead Press (with dumbbells or resistance band)

Stand with feet shoulder-width apart. Hold a dumbbell or handle of a resistance band in each hand with elbows bent at 90 degrees and pointing down and palms facing forward [1]. Press the dumbbells or resistance band handles up and in together over your head until they meet [2]. Lower the dumbbells or handles of the resistance band back along the same arc to the starting position and repeat for the prescribed number of reps.

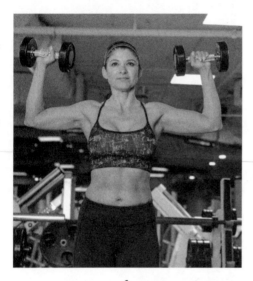

1

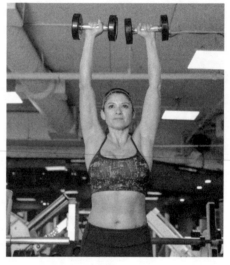

2

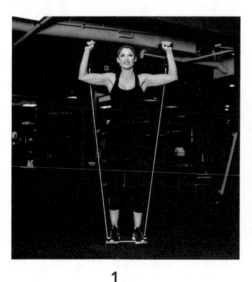

1

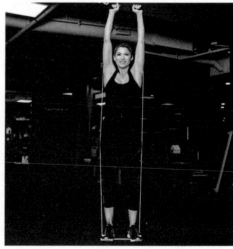

2

Stair Hops

Stand on your right leg at the bottom of a flight of stairs [1]. With your leg straight, hop up the stairs like a pogo stick, pushing off the ball of your foot [2]. Repeat for the prescribed number of reps before switching to the left leg.

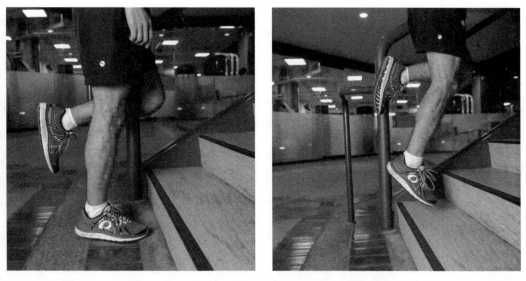

1   2

Short Circuit 3

Exercise	Reps
Dumbbell Chest Press	15–25
Wind Sprints	10
Overhead Press	15–25

Go immediately from one exercise to the next and do circuit 3 to 5 times, with no rest between circuits.

EXERCISE INSTRUCTIONS

Dumbbell Chest Press

Grab a dumbbell in each hand with an overhand grip and lie on your back on a flat bench with your feet flat on the floor.

Hold the dumbbells slightly greater than shoulder-width apart at the level of your chest with the palms of your hands facing each other and your elbows bent at 90 degrees with upper arms parallel to the floor [1]. In one curved motion, push the dumbbells upward by straightening your arms and bring the dumbbells in toward the midline of your chest while rotating your hands so that your palms face away from you as the ends of the dumbbells meet [2]. Lower the dumbbells back along the same arc to the level of your chest and repeat for the prescribed number of reps.

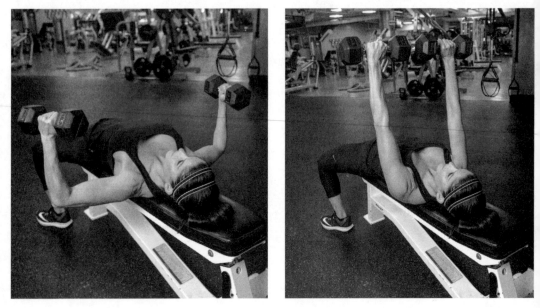

1   2

Wind Sprints

Place two cones about 50 feet apart from each other. Sprint from one cone to the other [1], bend down to tap the cone [2], and sprint back to the other cone. Repeat for the prescribed number of reps (each direction counts as one rep).

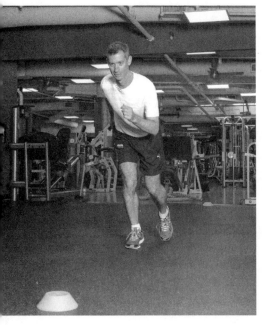
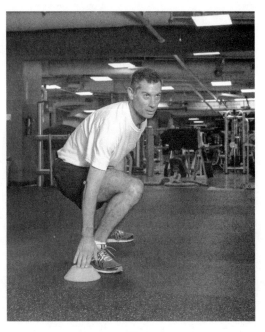

1 **2**

Overhead Press (with dumbbells or resistance band)

Stand with feet shoulder-width apart. Hold a dumbbell or handle of a resistance band in each hand with elbows bent at 90 degrees and pointing down and palms facing forward [1]. Press the dumbbells or resistance band handles up and in together over your head until they meet [2]. Lower the dumbbells or handles of the resistance band back along the same arc to the starting position and repeat for the prescribed number of reps.

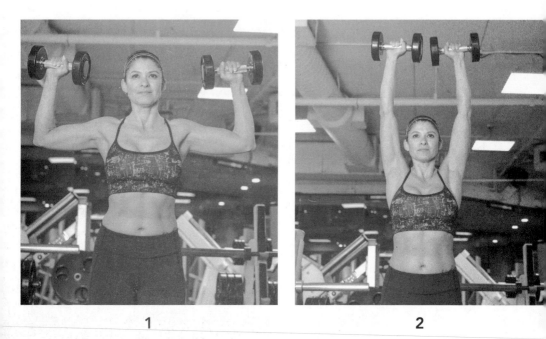

1   2

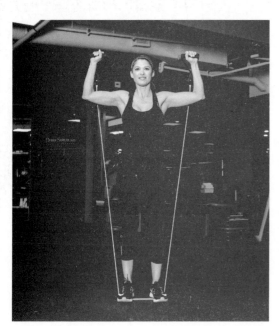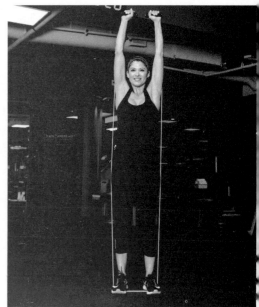

1   2

CHAPTER 4

MUSCULAR STRENGTH AND POWER WORKOUTS

In the early days of physical education, it was the strength of a muscle that garnered all of the attention. Tests of muscular strength have existed since at least the time of the ancient Olympics, when athletes were required to lift a ball of iron in order to qualify. In 1873, Dr. Dudley Sargent, a pioneer in physical education, initiated strength testing at Harvard University. It has since become an important tool in evaluating muscle characteristics.

Although many gym goers like to lift light weights, it is not enough for your muscles to endure; they must also be strong. Muscular endurance and muscular strength are different, albeit related, traits and are thus different components of physical fitness. Strong muscles are good-looking muscles.

To improve muscular strength, the intensity of your workouts must be high. You have to work at the maximum (or near maximum) ability of your muscles to produce force, and that can happen only if your muscles contract against a heavy resistance.

You can improve muscular strength two ways: (1) by making your muscles bigger (called *hypertrophy*) or (2) by increasing the ability of your central nervous system to "communicate" with your muscles by increasing the number of muscle fibers it recruits and increasing the frequency of recruiting signals it sends to your muscle fibers.

To get stronger by making muscles bigger, you need a strong enough stimulus to cause a substantial amount of muscle protein breakdown, which results in more muscle protein synthesis. To accomplish that, lift a relatively heavy weight—about 80 to 85 percent of the maximum you can lift just once—with enough recovery between sets to repeat the set at the prescribed intensity.

To get stronger by improving the neural communication to your muscles, lift very heavy weights—about 95 percent of the maximum you can lift just once—only 1 to 3 reps per set, with long recovery intervals between sets. For the neuromuscular workouts that use dumbbells, it's a good idea to work out with a buddy who can be your spotter since the weights are very heavy. When you train this way, you'll get a lot stronger without getting bigger muscles because the total number of reps—and therefore the total amount of protein breakdown—is low.

If you have ever tried to lift a heavy weight quickly, you'll notice that it's not possible. For a muscle to exert its maximum strength, it must produce force slowly. When you multiply muscular strength by the speed at which your muscles produce force, you get muscular power. For muscles to be powerful, they must be strong and they must be fast. To improve muscular power, lift a light weight quickly or use your own body weight with plyometrics.

This chapter gives you many options for muscular strength and power workouts using machines, free weights, and body weight so that you can do the workouts anywhere. All of the workouts in this chapter are designed to be completed in 14 minutes or less.

MUSCULAR HYPERTROPHY STRENGTH WORKOUTS

This series of workouts strengthens your muscles by increasing their definition and size. If you're a woman, don't worry—your muscles will not start to look like a man's, because you have much less testosterone to build muscle, so don't shy away from these workouts. The definition you'll create will make those men's heads turn! For all of these workouts, the intensity matters (they're only 14 minutes, after all!), so make sure you choose a weight that will fatigue your muscles for the prescribed rep range.

MACHINE WORKOUTS

Upper Body 1: Back & Biceps

Exercise	Sets	Reps	Intensity (% 1 rep max or RPE)	Recovery
Chin-Ups	3	5–8	80–85%	2:00
Seated Cable Row	3	5–8	80–85%	2:00
Biceps Preacher Curls	3	5–8	80–85%	2:00

EXERCISE INSTRUCTIONS

Chin-Ups

Stand on the platform of a weight-assisted chin-up machine. Grab the handles of the machine above your head with an underhand grip [1]. Pull yourself up until your chin reaches the height of your hands [2]. Lower yourself down to the starting position and repeat for the prescribed number of reps.

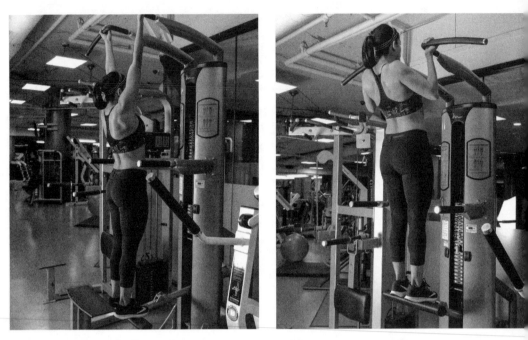

1   2

Seated Cable Row

Sit down on the machine and place your feet on the front platform with your knees slightly bent. Lean forward to grab the handles of the bar (use a V-bar that will keep your hands facing each other). Scoot back on the seat and pull the bar back with arms extended until your hips are at a 90-degree angle to your torso and your back is straight [1]. Using your back muscles, pull the handles of the bar toward your torso [2]. Slowly return to the starting position to lower the weight and repeat for the prescribed number of reps.

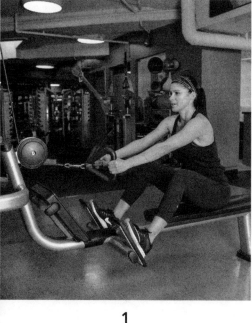
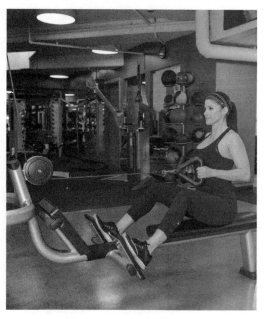

1   2

Biceps Preacher Curls

Sit on the seat of the machine and adjust the seat height so that you can comfortably extend your arms on the pad and your elbows are in line with the pivot point of the machine. Lay the back of your arms on the pad and grab the handles with an underhand grip [1]. Lift the weight by flexing your elbows, pulling your hands toward your shoulders [2]. Slowly return to the starting position to lower the weight and repeat for the prescribed number of reps.

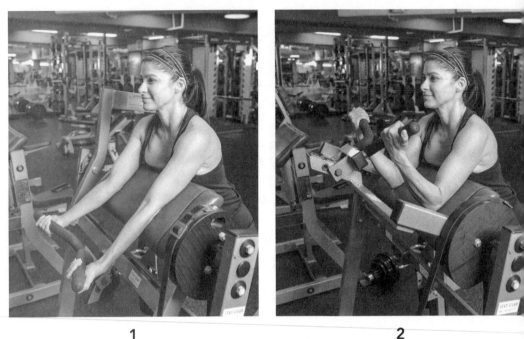

1   2

Upper Body 2: Chest, Shoulders, & Triceps

Exercise	Sets	Reps	Intensity (% 1 rep max or RPE)	Recovery
Chest Press	3	5–8	80–85%	2:00
Shoulder Press	3	5–8	80–85%	2:00
Triceps Pressdown	3	5–8	80–85%	2:00

EXERCISE INSTRUCTIONS

Chest Press

Sit with your back straight and flat against the back pad of the machine with feet flat on the floor. Grip the handles near your chest with an overhand grip [1]. Extend your arms to push the handles forward and up to lift the weight [2]. Slowly return to the starting position to lower the weight and repeat for the prescribed number of reps.

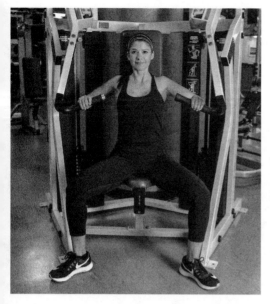
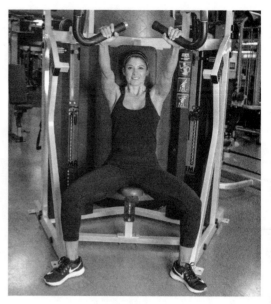

1   2

Shoulder Press

Sit down on the machine's seat with your back straight against the back pad. Adjust the seat height so that when you grab the handles, your hands are in line with your shoulders [1]. Push upward to lift the weight until your arms are fully extended [2]. Slowly return to the starting position to lower the weight and repeat for the prescribed number of reps.

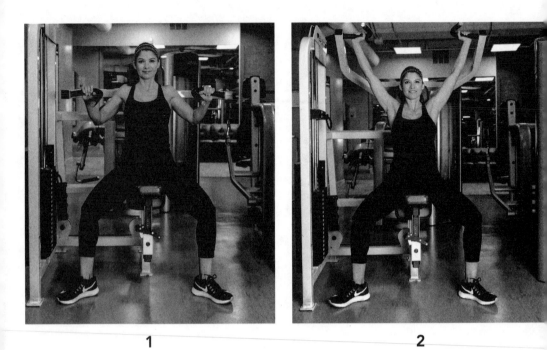

1 2

Triceps Pressdown

Attach a straight bar to a high pulley and grab the bar, using an overhand grip with your hands slightly less than shoulder-width apart. Stand with feet shoulder-width apart and your torso straight. Hold your upper arms close to your body with your elbows in to your sides and pointing down toward the floor [1]. Using your triceps, push the bar down until your arms are fully extended. Keep your upper arms stationary throughout the movement and hold them next to your torso [2]. Slowly return to the starting position to lower the weight and repeat for the prescribed number of reps.

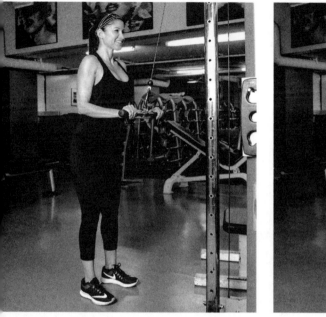
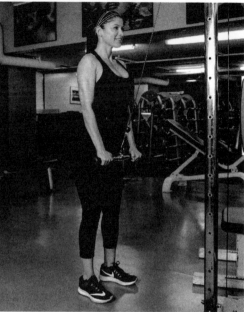

1   2

Lower Body 1: Quads & Calves

Exercise	Sets	Reps	Intensity (% 1 rep max or RPE)	Recovery
Squats (Smith machine)	3	5–8	80–85%	2:00
Calf Press	3	5–8	80–85%	2:00
Leg Press	3	5–8	80–85%	2:00

EXERCISE INSTRUCTIONS

Squats (Smith machine)

Set the bar on the Smith machine to the height of your shoulders. Place any extra weight on the bar that you need to meet the prescribed intensity. With feet shoulder-width or slightly greater than shoulder-width apart, stand in front of the barbell. Place the barbell across the back of your shoulders below your neck and grab the barbell from behind with a grip slightly greater than shoulder-width. Lift the barbell from the rack so it rests on your shoulders and upper back [1]. Keeping your back straight, bend your knees and squat down until your thighs are parallel to the floor. Move your hips back as if you're going to sit in a chair [2]. Push against the floor to return to the starting position and repeat for the prescribed number of reps.

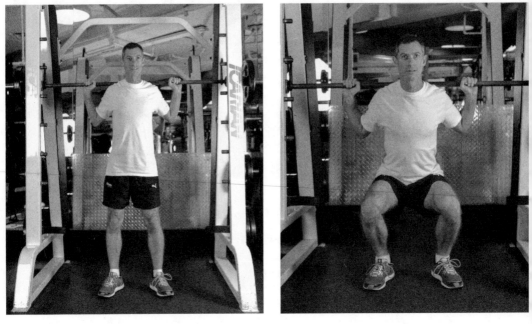

1   2

Calf Press

Sit on the seat of a seated calf press machine and place your toes and the balls of your feet on the platform in front of you with your feet shoulder-width apart, legs slightly bent, and your back against the seat cushion. Grab the side handles of the machine for support [1]. Push against the platform with the balls of your feet to lift the weight [2]. Slowly return to the starting position and repeat for the prescribed number of reps.

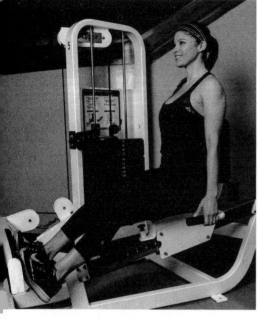

1

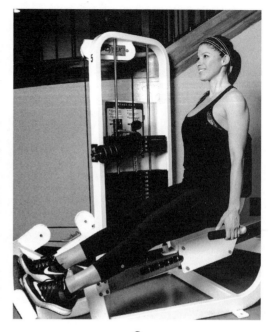

2

Leg Press

Sit on the leg press machine with your feet shoulder-width apart on the platform and your back flat against the back pad. Adjust the seat position so that your knees are bent at 90 degrees. Grab the side handles for support [1]. Lift the weight by pressing your feet against the platform and straightening your legs until just before your legs are completely straight [2]. Throughout the motion, keep your legs parallel to one another. Slowly return to the starting position to lower the weight and repeat for the prescribed number of reps.

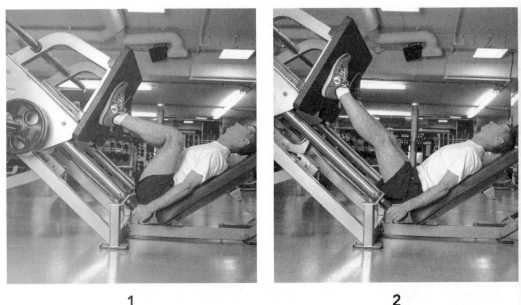

1 2

Lower Body 2: Hamstrings & Glutes

Exercise	Sets	Reps	Intensity (% 1 rep max or RPE)	Recovery
Leg Curl	3	5–8	80–85%	2:00
Hip Extension	3	5–8	80–85%	2:00
Low-Cable Deadlift	3	5–8	80–85%	2:00

EXERCISE INSTRUCTIONS

Leg Curl

Lie facedown on the leg curl machine with your hips flat against the bench, your legs straight, and the leg pad on the back of your legs, just below your calves. Adjust the length of the lever and your position on the pad so that when you lie down, your knees are in line with the pivot point of the machine. Grab the handles of the machine for support [1]. Curl your legs up until your heels come close to your butt [2]. Slowly return to the starting position to lower the weight and repeat for the prescribed number of reps.

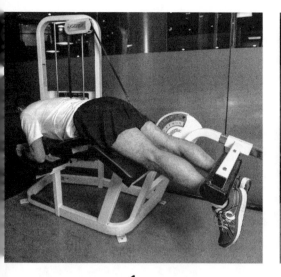

1

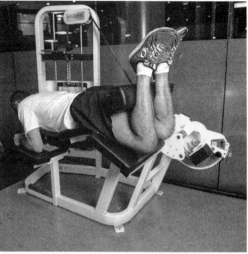

2

Hip Extension

Hook an ankle cuff to a low cable pulley and attach the cuff to your ankle. Stand about two feet from the machine, lean slightly forward, and grab the frame for support [1]. Squeeze your glutes and extend the cuffed leg backward, keeping the leg straight [2]. Slowly return to the starting position and repeat for the prescribed number of reps before switching to the other leg.

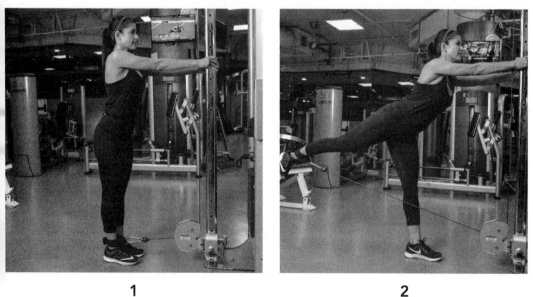

1   2

Low-Cable Deadlift

Attach a straight bar to the cable machine and set it to the lowest setting. Grab the bar with an overhand, shoulder-width grip and step back about two steps. Stand with your feet shoulder-width apart, legs straight or slightly bent, and bend over from your waist with your back straight [1]. Lift the bar by raising your torso to stand up straight, keeping your legs and back straight [2]. Slowly lower the bar to the starting position and repeat for the prescribed number of reps.

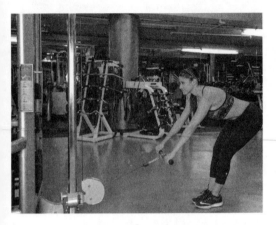

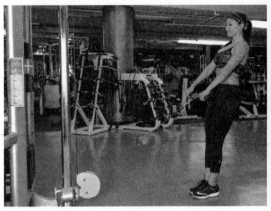

1   2

Upper Body Strength Pyramid

Exercise	Sets	Reps	Intensity (% 1 rep max or RPE)	Recovery
Chest Press	1 / 2 / 3	10 / 8 / 6	75–80 / 80–85 / 85–90%	1:00
Seated Cable Row	1 / 2 / 3	10 / 8 / 6	75–80 / 80–85 / 85–90%	1:00
Biceps Preacher Curls	1 / 2 / 3	10 / 8 / 6	75–80 / 80–85 / 85–90%	1:00
Triceps Pressdown	1 / 2 / 3	10 / 8 / 6	75–80 / 80–85 / 85–90%	1:00

Increase the amount of weight by 5 to 10 pounds as you decrease the number of reps in each set.

EXERCISE INSTRUCTIONS

Chest Press

Sit with your back straight and flat against the back pad of the machine with feet flat on the floor. Grip the handles near your chest with an overhand grip [1]. Extend your arms to push the handles forward and up to lift the weight [2]. Slowly return to the starting position to lower the weight and repeat for the prescribed number of reps.

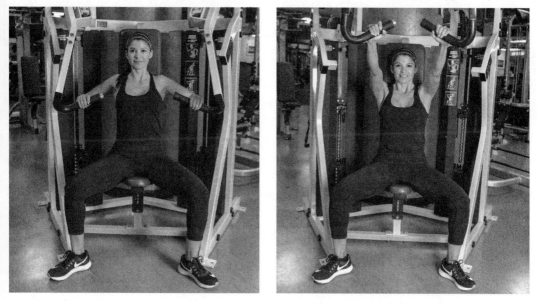

1   2

Seated Cable Row

Sit down on the machine and place your feet on the front platform with your knees slightly bent. Lean forward to grab the handles of the bar (use a V-bar that will keep your hands facing each other). Scoot back on the seat and pull the bar back with arms extended until your hips are at a 90-degree angle to your torso and your back is straight [1]. Using your back muscles, pull the handles of the bar toward your torso [2]. Slowly return to the starting position to lower the weight and repeat for the prescribed number of reps.

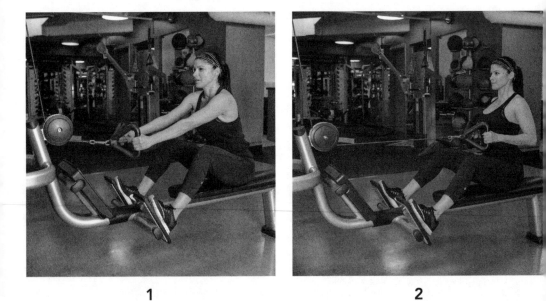

1   **2**

Biceps Preacher Curls

Sit on the seat of the machine and adjust the seat height so that you can comfortably extend your arms on the pad and your elbows are in line with the pivot point of the machine. Lay the back of your arms on the pad and grab the handles with an underhand grip [1]. Lift the weight by flexing your elbows, pulling your hands toward your shoulders [2]. Slowly return to the starting position to lower the weight and repeat for the prescribed number of reps.

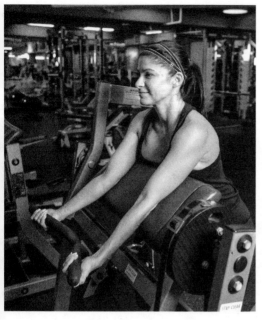
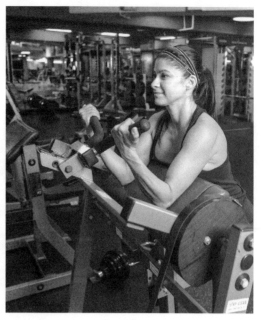

1   2

Triceps Pressdown

Attach a straight bar to a high pulley and grab the bar, using an overhand grip with your hands slightly less than shoulder-width apart. Stand with feet shoulder-width apart and your torso straight. Hold your upper arms close to your body with your elbows in to your sides and pointing down toward the floor [1]. Using your triceps, push the bar down until your arms are fully extended. Keep your upper arms stationary throughout the movement and hold them next to your torso [2]. Slowly return to the starting position to lower the weight and repeat for the prescribed number of reps.

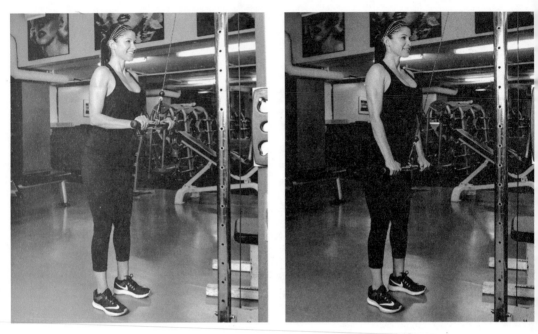

1   2

Lower Body Strength Pyramid

Exercise	Sets	Reps	Intensity (% 1 rep max or RPE)	Recovery
Squats (Smith machine)	1 / 2 / 3	10 / 8 / 6	75–80 / 80–85 / 85–90%	1:00
Leg Curl	1 / 2 / 3	10 / 8 / 6	75–80 / 80–85 / 85–90%	1:00
Leg Extension	1 / 2 / 3	10 / 8 / 6	75–80 / 80–85 / 85–90%	1:00
Leg Press	1 / 2 / 3	10 / 8 / 6	75–80 / 80–85 / 85–90%	1:00

Increase the amount of weight by 5 to 10 pounds as you decrease the number of reps in each set.

EXERCISE INSTRUCTIONS

Squats (Smith machine)

Set the bar on the Smith machine to the height of your shoulders. Place any extra weight on the bar that you need to meet the prescribed intensity. With feet shoulder-width or slightly greater than shoulder-width apart, stand in front of the barbell. Place the barbell across the back of your shoulders below your neck and grab the barbell from behind with a grip slightly greater than shoulder-width. Lift the barbell from the rack so it rests on your shoulders and upper back [1]. Keeping your back straight, bend your knees and squat down until your thighs are parallel to the floor. Move your hips back as if you're going to sit in a chair [2]. Push against the floor to return to the starting position and repeat for the prescribed number of reps.

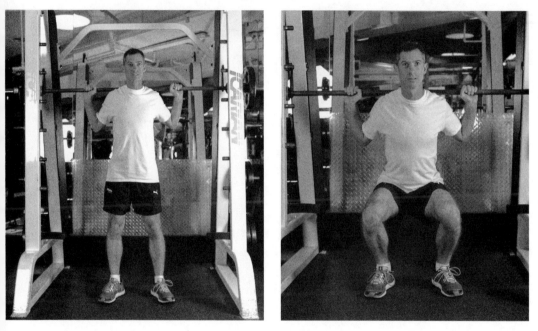

1   2

Leg Curl

Lie facedown on the leg curl machine with your hips flat against the bench, your legs straight, and the leg pad on the back of your legs, just below your calves. Adjust the length of the lever and your position on the pad so that when you lie down, your knees are in line with the pivot point of the machine. Grab the handles of the machine for support [1]. Curl your legs up until your heels come close to your butt [2]. Slowly return to the starting position to lower the weight and repeat for the prescribed number of reps.

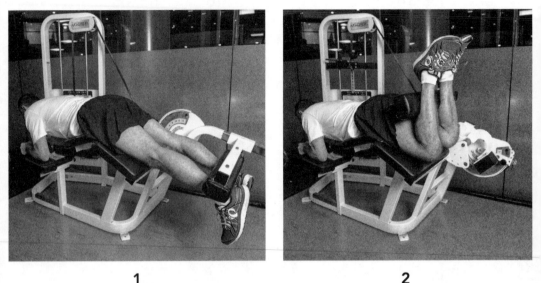

1   2

Leg Extension

Sit on the leg extension machine with your legs under the circular pad and your feet pointed forward. Adjust the length of the lever and your position in the seat so that your knees form a 90-degree angle and are in line with the pivot point of the machine. Adjust the pad so it sits at ankle height. Grab the side handles of the machine for support [1]. Using your quadriceps, extend your legs until they are straight [2]. Slowly return to the starting position to lower the weight and repeat for the prescribed number of reps.

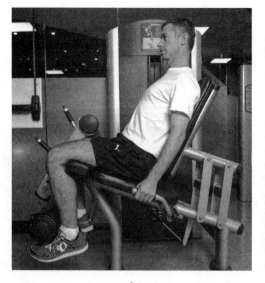
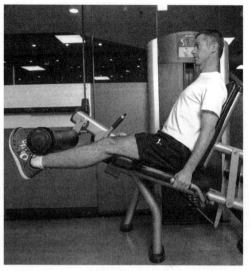

1
2

Leg Press

Sit on the leg press machine with your feet shoulder-width apart on the platform and your back flat against the back pad. Adjust the seat position so that your knees are bent at 90 degrees. Grab the side handles for support [1]. Lift the weight by pressing your feet against the platform and straightening your legs until just before your legs are completely straight [2]. Throughout the motion, keep your legs parallel to one another. Slowly return to the starting position to lower the weight and repeat for the prescribed number of reps.

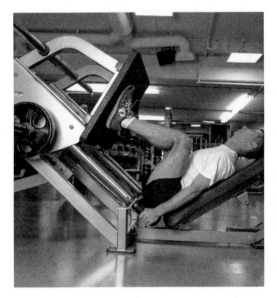

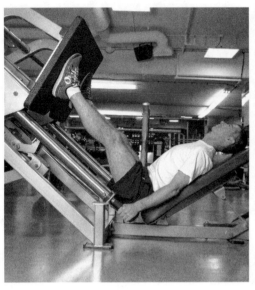

1   2

Upper Body Drop Sets

Exercise	Sets	Reps	Intensity (% 1 rep max or RPE)
Chest Press	3	10	80–85 / 75–80 / 70–75%
Chin-Ups	3	10	80–85 / 75–80 / 70–75%
Seated Cable Row	3	10	80–85 / 75–80 / 70–75%
Triceps Pressdown	3	10	80–85 / 75–80 / 70–75%

Decrease the amount of weight after the first set by 5 to 10 pounds and immediately do the next set of 10 reps. Then drop the weight again by another 5 to 10 pounds and immediately do the third set.

EXERCISE INSTRUCTIONS

Chest Press

Sit with your back straight and flat against the back pad of the machine with feet flat on the floor. Grip the handles near your chest with an overhand grip [1]. Extend your arms to push the handles forward and up to lift the weight [2]. Slowly return to the starting position to lower the weight and repeat for the prescribed number of reps.

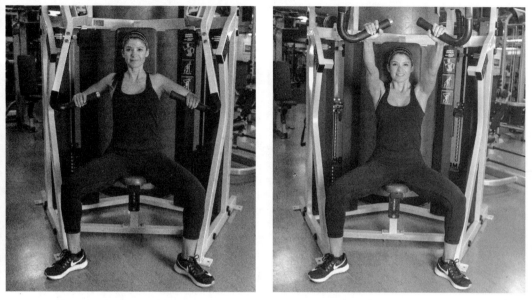

1   2

Chin-Ups

Stand on the platform of a weight-assisted chin-up machine. Grab the handles of the machine above your head with an underhand grip [1]. Pull yourself up until your chin reaches the height of your hands [2]. Lower yourself down to the starting position and repeat for the prescribed number of reps.

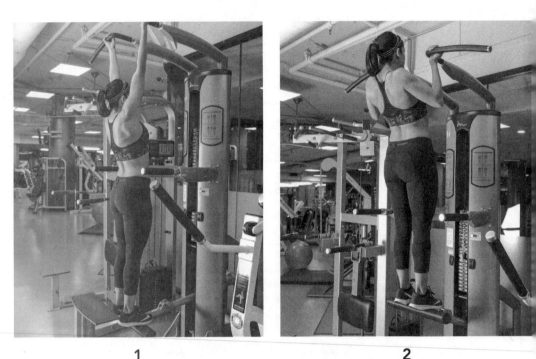

1   2

Seated Cable Row

Sit down on the machine and place your feet on the front platform with your knees slightly bent. Lean forward to grab the handles of the bar (use a V-bar that will keep your hands facing each other). Scoot back on the seat and pull the bar back with arms extended until your hips are at a 90-degree angle to your torso and your back is straight [1]. Using your back muscles, pull the handles of the bar toward your torso [2]. Slowly return to the starting position to lower the weight and repeat for the prescribed number of reps.

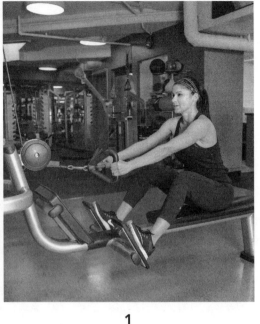

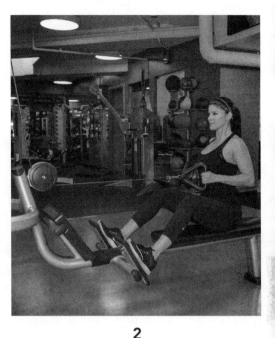

1   2

Triceps Pressdown

Attach a straight bar to a high pulley and grab the bar, using an overhand grip with your hands slightly less than shoulder-width apart. Stand with feet shoulder-width apart and your torso straight. Hold your upper arms close to your body with your elbows in to your sides and pointing down toward the floor [1]. Using your triceps, push the bar down until your arms are fully extended. Keep your upper arms stationary throughout the movement and hold them next to your torso [2]. Slowly return to the starting position to lower the weight and repeat for the prescribed number of reps.

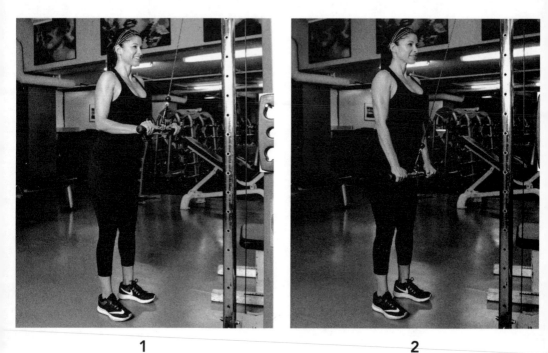

1   2

Lower Body Drop Sets

Exercise	Sets	Reps	Intensity (% 1 rep max or RPE)
Squats (Smith machine)	3	10	80–85 / 75–80 / 70–75%
Leg Curl	3	10	80–85 / 75–80 / 70–75%
Leg Extension	3	10	80–85 / 75–80 / 70–75%
Leg Press	3	10	80–85 / 75–80 / 70–75%

Decrease the amount of weight after the first set by 5 to 10 pounds and immediately do the next set of 10 reps. Then drop the weight again by another 5 to 10 pounds and immediately do the third set.

EXERCISE INSTRUCTIONS

Squats (Smith machine)

Set the bar on the Smith machine to the height of your shoulders. Place any extra weight on the bar that you need to meet the prescribed intensity. With feet shoulder-width or slightly greater than shoulder-width apart, stand in front of the barbell. Place the barbell across the back of your shoulders below your neck and grab the barbell from behind with a grip slightly greater than shoulder-width. Lift the barbell from the rack so it rests on your shoulders and upper back [1]. Keeping your back straight, bend your knees and squat down until your thighs are parallel to the floor. Move your hips back as if you're going to sit in a chair [2]. Push against the floor to return to the starting position and repeat for the prescribed number of reps.

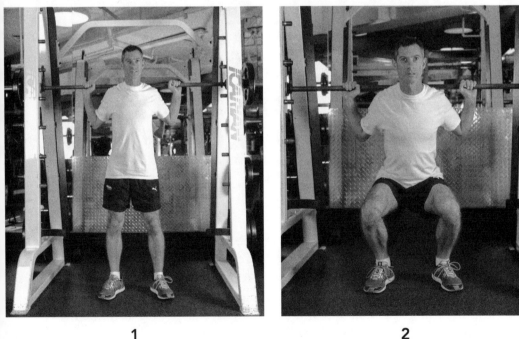

1   2

Leg Curl

Lie facedown on the leg curl machine with your hips flat against the bench, your legs straight, and the leg pad on the back of your legs, just below your calves. Adjust the length of the lever and your position on the pad so that when you lie down, your knees are in line with the pivot point of the machine. Grab the handles of the machine for support [1]. Curl your legs up until your heels come close to your butt [2]. Slowly return to the starting position to lower the weight and repeat for the prescribed number of reps.

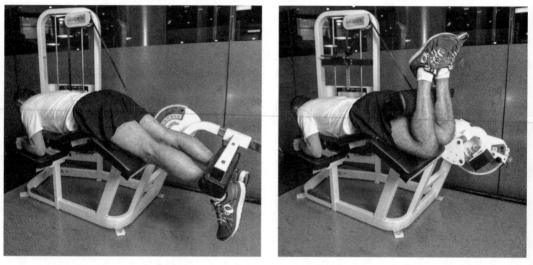

1   2

Leg Extension

Sit on the leg extension machine with your legs under the circular pad and your feet pointed forward. Adjust the length of the lever and your position in the seat so that your knees form a 90-degree angle and are in line with the pivot point of the machine. Adjust the pad so it sits just above your ankles. Grab the side handles of the machine for support [1]. Using your quadriceps, extend your legs until they are straight [2]. Slowly return to the starting position to lower the weight and repeat for the prescribed number of reps.

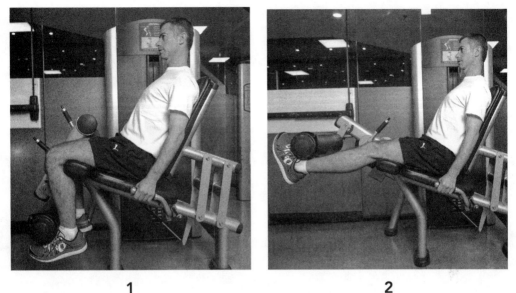

1 2

Leg Press

Sit on the leg press machine with your feet shoulder-width apart on the platform and your back flat against the back pad. Adjust the seat position so that your knees are bent at 90 degrees. Grab the side handles for support [1]. Lift the weight by pressing your feet against the platform and straightening your legs until just before your legs are completely straight [2]. Throughout the motion, keep your legs parallel to one another. Slowly return to the starting position to lower the weight and repeat for the prescribed number of reps.

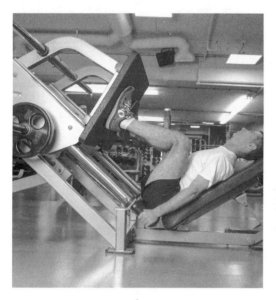

1

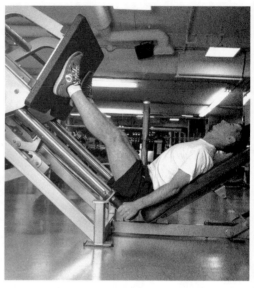

2

Total Body Machine Workout

Exercise	Sets	Reps	Intensity (% 1 rep max or RPE)
Leg Press	1	as many as possible	80–85%
Chin-Ups	1	as many as possible	80–85%
Leg Curl	1	as many as possible	80–85%
Chest Press	1	as many as possible	80–85%
Hip Extension	1	as many as possible	80–85%
Shoulder Press	1	as many as possible	80–85%
Calf Press	1	as many as possible	80–85%
Seated Cable Row	1	as many as possible	80–85%

Exercises alternate between lower body and upper body and progress from bigger muscles to smaller muscles. Move immediately from one exercise to the next.

EXERCISE INSTRUCTIONS

Leg Press

Sit on the leg press machine with your feet shoulder-width apart on the platform and your back flat against the back pad. Adjust the seat position so that your knees are bent at 90 degrees. Grab the side handles for support [1]. Lift the weight by pressing your feet against the platform and straightening your legs until just before your legs are completely straight [2]. Throughout the motion, keep your legs parallel to one another. Slowly return to the starting position to lower the weight and repeat for the prescribed number of reps.

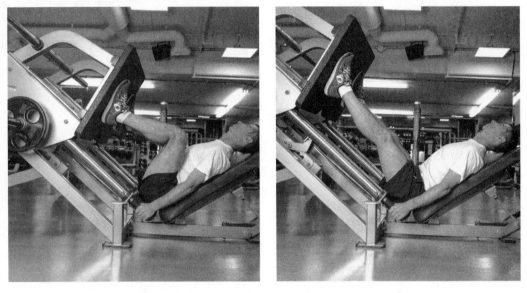

1   2

Chin-Ups

Stand on the platform of a weight-assisted chin-up machine. Grab the handles of the machine above your head with an underhand grip [1]. Pull yourself up until your chin reaches the height of your hands [2]. Lower yourself down to the starting position and repeat for the prescribed number of reps.

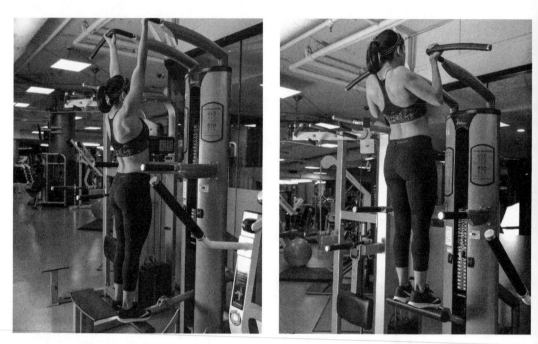

1   2

Leg Curl

Lie facedown on the leg curl machine with your hips flat against the bench, your legs straight, and the leg pad on the back of your legs, just below your calves. Adjust the length of the lever and your position on the pad so that when you lie down, your knees are in line with the pivot point of the machine. Grab the handles of the machine for support [1]. Curl your legs up until your heels come close to your butt [2]. Slowly return to the starting position to lower the weight and repeat for the prescribed number of reps.

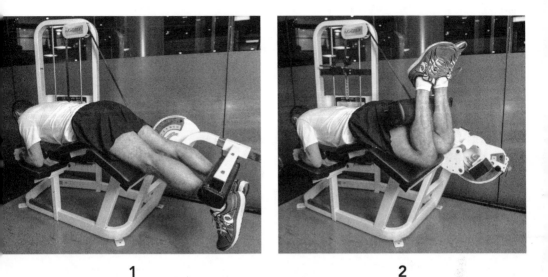

1   2

Chest Press

Sit with your back straight and flat against the back pad of the machine with feet flat on the floor. Grip the handles near your chest with an overhand grip [1]. Extend your arms to push the handles forward and up to lift the weight [2]. Slowly return to the starting position to lower the weight and repeat for the prescribed number of reps.

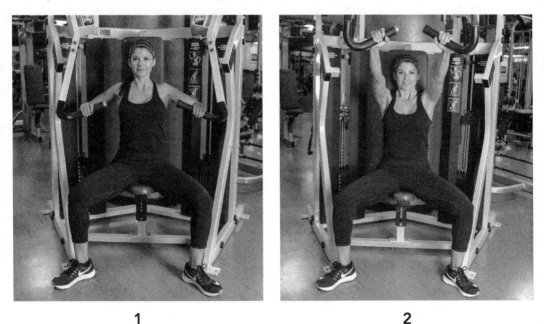

1   2

Hip Extension

Hook an ankle cuff to a low cable pulley and attach the cuff to your ankle. Stand about two feet from the machine, lean slightly forward, and grab the frame for support [1]. Squeeze your glutes and extend the cuffed leg backward, keeping the leg straight [2]. Slowly return to the starting position and repeat for the prescribed number of reps before switching to the other leg.

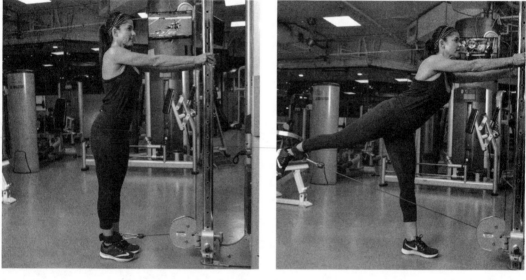

1   2

Shoulder Press

Sit down on the machine's seat with your back straight against the back pad. Adjust the seat height so that when you grab the handles, your hands are in line with your shoulders [1]. Push upward to lift the weight until your arms are fully extended [2]. Slowly return to the starting position to lower the weight and repeat for the prescribed number of reps.

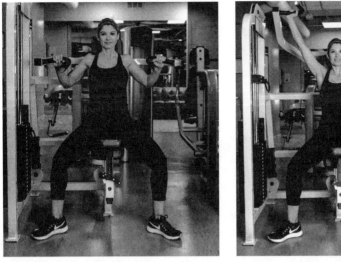
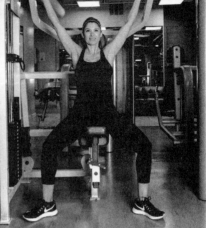

1   2

Calf Press

Sit on the seat of a seated calf press machine and place your toes and the balls of your feet on the platform in front of you with your feet shoulder-width apart, legs slightly bent, and your back against the seat cushion. Grab the side handles of the machine for support [1]. Push against the platform with the balls of your feet to lift the weight [2]. Slowly return to the starting position and repeat for the prescribed number of reps.

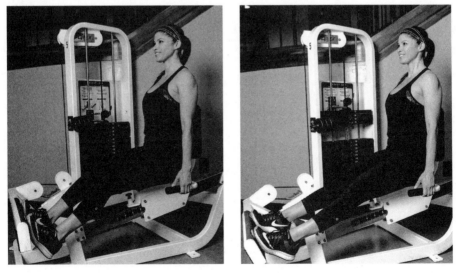

1   2

Seated Cable Row

Sit down on the machine and place your feet on the front platform with your knees slightly bent. Lean forward to grab the handles of the bar (use a V-bar that will keep your hands facing each other). Scoot back on the seat and pull the bar back with arms extended until your hips are at a 90-degree angle to your torso and your back is straight [1]. Using your back muscles, pull the handles of the bar toward your torso [2]. Slowly return to the starting position to lower the weight and repeat for the prescribed number of reps.

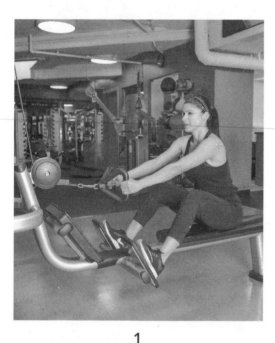

1

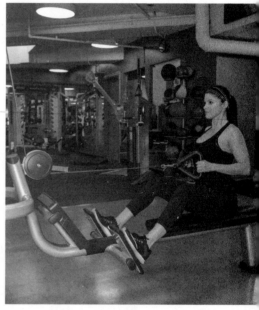

2

DUMBBELL WORKOUTS

Upper Body 1: Back & Biceps

Exercise	Sets	Reps	Intensity (% 1 rep max or RPE)	Recovery
Dumbbell Row	3	5–8	80–85%	2:00
Dumbbell Reverse Flys	3	5–8	80–85%	2:00
Dumbbell Biceps Curls	3	5–8	80–85%	2:00

EXERCISE INSTRUCTIONS

Dumbbell Row

Stand with feet shoulder-width apart with knees slightly bent and hold a dumbbell in each hand with palms facing each other. Keeping your back straight, bend over at the waist until your back is almost parallel to the floor. The dumbbells should hang directly in front of you as your arms hang perpendicular to the floor and your torso [1]. While keeping your torso stationary, use your shoulder muscles to lift the dumbbells, keeping your elbows close to your body [2]. Slowly lower the dumbbells to the starting position and repeat for the prescribed number of reps.

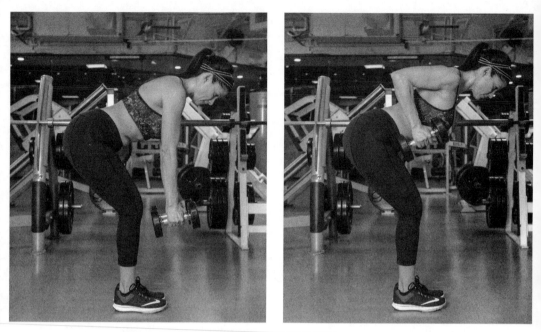

1

2

Dumbbell Reverse Flys

Grab a dumbbell in each hand with an overhand grip and palms facing each other and stand with feet shoulder-width apart. Slightly bend your knees and lean forward from your hips with your back straight. Hold the dumbbells with your arms slightly bent [1]. Raise your arms out to your sides like a fly opening its wings until your elbows are slightly higher than your shoulders [2]. Lower the dumbbells to the starting position and repeat for the prescribed number of reps. You can also do this exercise on an incline bench with your torso flat against the bench [3 & 4].

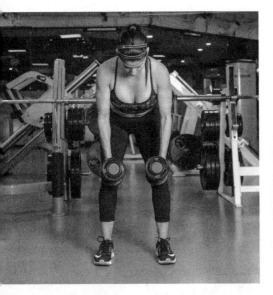

1

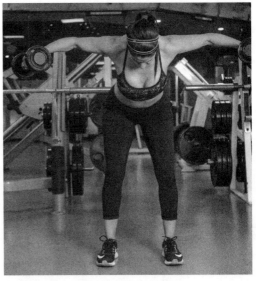

2

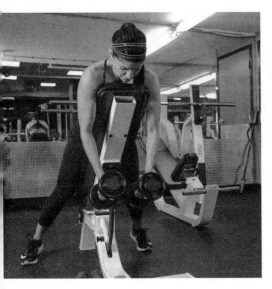

3

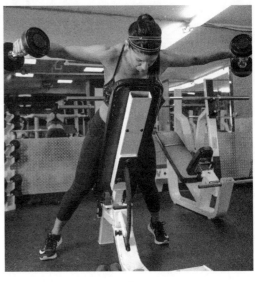

4

Dumbbell Biceps Curls

Stand with feet shoulder-width apart and your back straight. Hold a dumbbell in each hand with your arms by your sides. Keep your elbows close to your body [1]. Lift the dumbbells by bending your elbows and rotate your hands so that your palms face up as the dumbbells reach your shoulders [2]. Lower the dumbbells to the starting position and repeat for the prescribed number of reps.

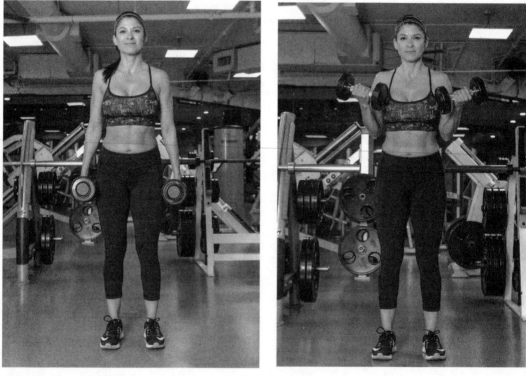

1   2

Upper Body 2: Chest, Shoulders, & Triceps

Exercise	Sets	Reps	Intensity (% 1 rep max or RPE)	Recovery
Dumbbell Chest Press	3	5–8	80–85%	2:00
Dumbbell Overhead Press	3	5–8	80–85%	2:00
Dumbbell Triceps Kickback	3	5–8	80–85%	2:00

EXERCISE INSTRUCTIONS

Dumbbell Chest Press

Grab a dumbbell in each hand with an overhand grip and lie on your back on a flat bench with your feet flat on the floor. Hold the dumbbells slightly greater than shoulder-width apart at the level of your chest with the palms of your hands facing each other and your elbows bent at 90 degrees with upper arms parallel to the floor [1]. In one curved motion, push the dumbbells upward by straightening your arms and bring the dumbbells in toward the midline of your chest while rotating your hands so that your palms face away from you as the ends of the dumbbells meet [2]. Lower the dumbbells back along the same arc to the level of your chest and repeat for the prescribed number of reps.

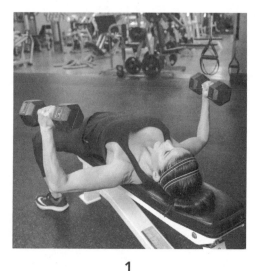

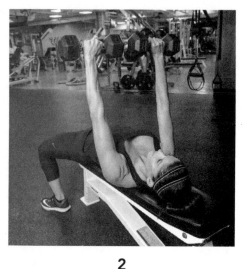

1

2

Dumbbell Overhead Press

Stand with feet shoulder-width apart. Hold a dumbbell in each hand with elbows bent at 90 degrees and pointing down and palms facing forward [1]. Press the dumbbells up and in together over your head [2]. Lower the dumbbells back along the same arc to the starting position, keeping the weight balanced over your elbows, and repeat for the prescribed number of reps.

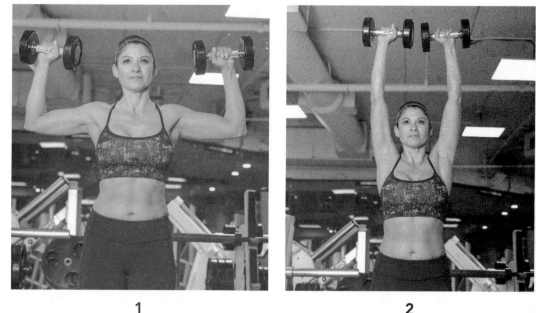

1

2

14-MINUTE METABOLIC WORKOUTS

Dumbbell Triceps Kickback

Kneel on a bench with your left leg and place your left arm on the bench for support. Hold a dumbbell in your right hand with your upper arm parallel to the floor and your elbow bent at 90 degrees [1]. Extend your arm at the elbow until your arm is straight. Only your forearm should move [2]. Slowly return to the starting position and repeat for the prescribed number of reps before switching to the left arm.

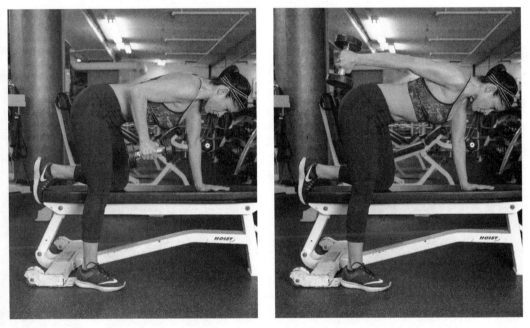

1   2

Lower Body 1: Quads & Calves

Exercise	Sets	Reps	Intensity (% 1 rep max or RPE)	Recovery
Dumbbell Squats	3	5–8	80–85%	2:00
Dumbbell Calf Raises	3	5–8	80–85%	2:00
Dumbbell Step-Ups	3	5–8	80–85%	2:00

EXERCISE INSTRUCTIONS

Dumbbell Squats

Stand with feet shoulder-width or slightly wider than shoulder-width apart with a dumbbell in each hand and arms fully extended with palms facing the side of your legs [1]. Keeping your back straight, bend your knees and squat down until your thighs are parallel to the floor. Move your hips back as if you're going to sit in a chair [2]. Push against the floor to return to the starting position and repeat for the prescribed number of reps.

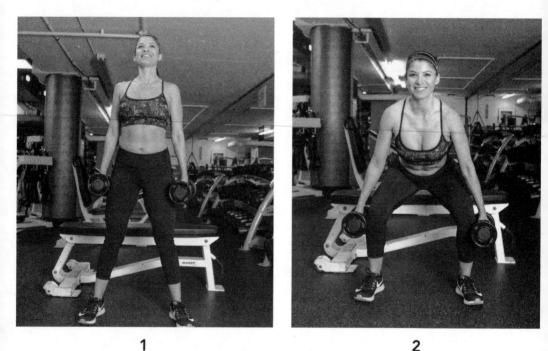

1   2

Dumbbell Calf Raises

Hold a dumbbell in each hand and stand with legs together, with one foot off the ground [1]. With the other foot, push against the ground with the ball of your foot to raise yourself up [2]. Slowly return to the starting position and repeat for the prescribed number of reps.

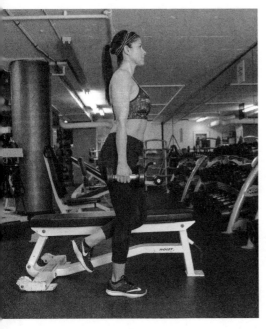
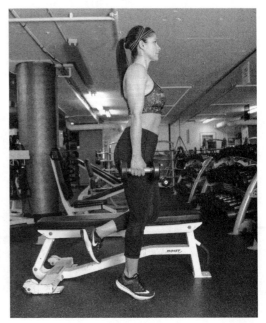

1

2

Dumbbell Step-Ups

Stand behind a bench or other elevated platform with a dumbbell in each hand and your palms facing the side of your legs [1]. Step up onto the bench with your right leg [2] and then place your left foot on the bench [3]. Step down with your left leg to return to the starting position and repeat for the prescribed number of reps before switching to leading with the left leg.

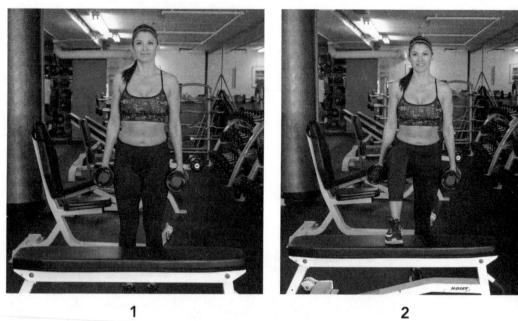

1

2

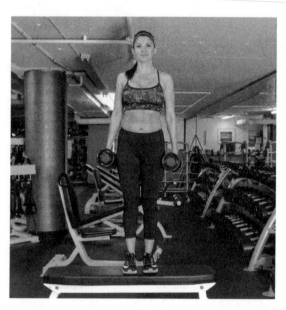

3

14-MINUTE METABOLIC WORKOUTS

Lower Body 2: Hamstrings, Glutes, & Inner Thighs

Exercise	Sets	Reps	Intensity (% 1 rep max or RPE)	Recovery
Dumbbell Deadlift	3	5–8	80–85%	2:00
Dumbbell Side Lunges	3	5–8	80–85%	2:00
Dumbbell Plié Squats	3	5–8	80–85%	2:00

EXERCISE INSTRUCTIONS

Dumbbell Deadlift

Hold a dumbbell in each hand by your sides at arm's length and stand with your feet shoulder-width apart [1]. Keeping your back and legs straight, bend over at the waist to lower the dumbbells until your back is parallel to the floor. As you bend over, you should feel a stretch in your hamstrings [2]. Keeping your back and legs straight, stand upright to return to the starting position and repeat for the prescribed number of reps.

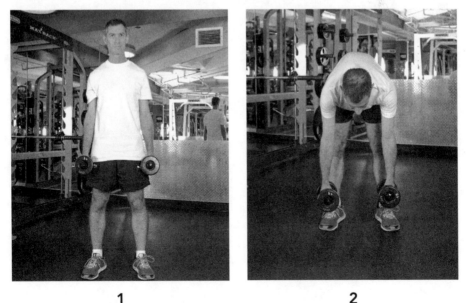

1   2

Dumbbell Side Lunges

Hold a dumbbell in each hand in front of you, with your palms facing each other, and stand with your feet shoulder-width apart [1]. Take a big lateral step out to your left side and lower yourself into a squat, keeping your right leg straight [2]. Push back up with your left leg to return to the starting position and repeat for the prescribed number of reps before switching to the right leg.

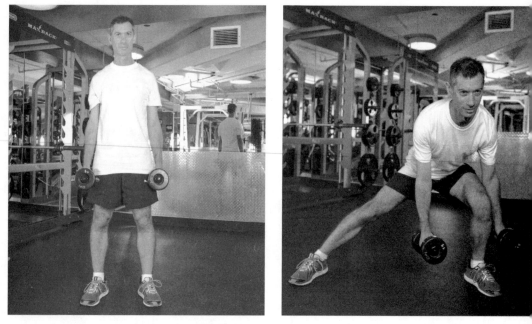

1   2

Dumbbell Plié Squats

Stand with feet slightly greater than shoulder-width apart and toes turned out about 45 degrees. Hold a dumbbell vertically with both hands between your legs [1]. Keeping your back straight, squat down until your thighs are parallel to the floor [2]. Push through your feet to stand up to return to the starting position and repeat for the prescribed number of reps.

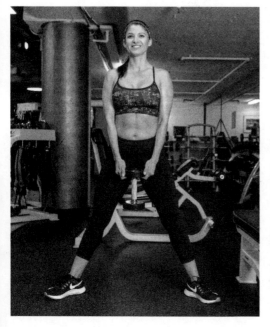
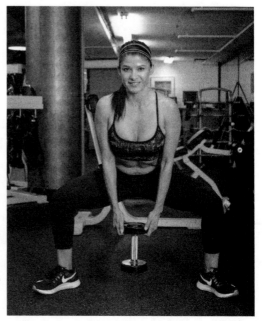

1   2

Total Body Dumbbell Workout

Exercise	Sets	Reps	Intensity (% 1 rep max or RPE)
Dumbbell Squats	1	as many as possible	80–85%
Dumbbell Chest Press	1	as many as possible	80–85%
Dumbbell Lunges	1	as many as possible	80–85%
Dumbbell Reverse Flys	1	as many as possible	80–85%
Dumbbell Deadlift	1	as many as possible	80–85%
Dumbbell Row	1	as many as possible	80–85%
Dumbbell Calf Raises	1	as many as possible	80–85%
Dumbbell Biceps Curls	1	as many as possible	80–85%

Exercises alternate between lower body and upper body and progress from bigger muscles to smaller muscles. Move immediately from one exercise to the next.

Dumbbell Squats

Stand with feet shoulder-width or slightly wider than shoulder-width apart with a dumbbell in each hand and arms fully extended with palms facing the side of your legs [1]. Keeping your back straight, bend your knees and squat down until your thighs are parallel to the floor. Move your hips back as if you're going to sit in a chair [2]. Push against the floor to return to the starting position and repeat for the prescribed number of reps.

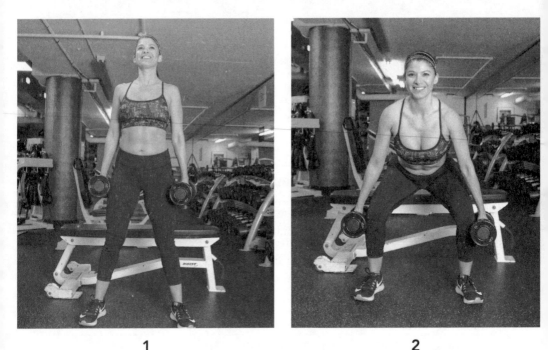

1   2

Dumbbell Chest Press

Grab a dumbbell in each hand with an overhand grip and lie on your back on a flat bench with your feet flat on the floor. Hold the dumbbells slightly greater than shoulder-width apart at the level of your chest with the palms of your hands facing each other and your elbows bent at 90 degrees with upper arms parallel to the floor [1]. In one curved motion, push the dumbbells upward by straightening your arms and bring the dumbbells in toward the midline of your chest while rotating your hands so that your palms face away from you as the ends of the dumbbells meet [2]. Lower the dumbbells back along the same arc to the level of your chest and repeat for the prescribed number of reps.

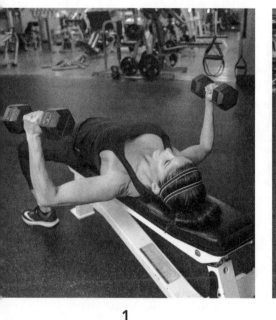 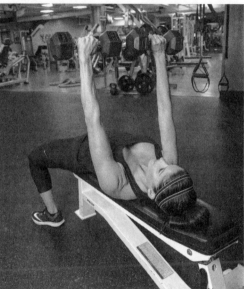

1   2

Dumbbell Lunges

Stand with your torso upright, holding a dumbbell in each hand by your sides [1]. Step forward about two feet with your right leg and lower yourself down into the lunge while keeping your torso upright. Keep your right knee above your toes as you lunge forward and keep your right shin perpendicular to the ground [2]. Push yourself back up and lunge forward with your left leg. Repeat for the prescribed number of reps.

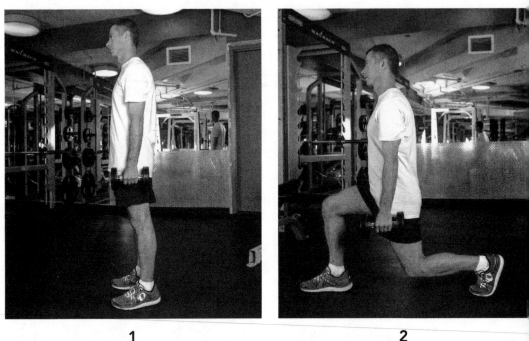

1   2

Dumbbell Reverse Flys

Grab a dumbbell in each hand with an overhand grip and palms facing each other and stand with feet shoulder-width apart. Slightly bend your knees and lean forward from your hips with your back straight. Hold the dumbbells with your arms slightly bent [1]. Raise your arms out to your sides like a fly opening its wings until your elbows are slightly higher than your shoulders [2]. Lower the dumbbells to the starting position and repeat for the prescribed number of reps. You can also do this exercise on an incline bench with your torso flat against the bench [3 & 4].

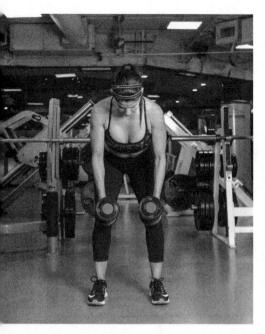

1

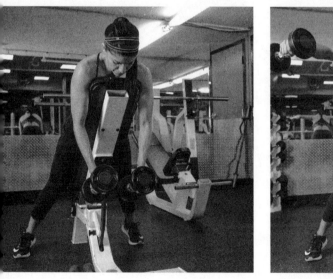

2

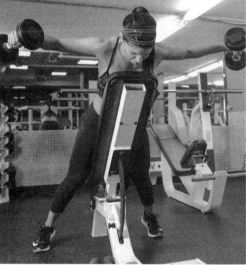

3

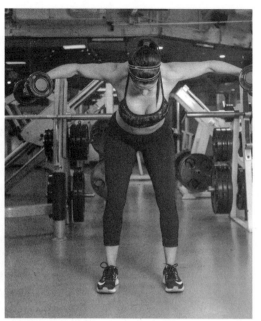

4

Dumbbell Deadlift

Hold a dumbbell in each hand by your sides at arm's length and stand with your feet shoulder-width apart [1]. Keeping your back and legs straight, bend over at the waist to lower the dumbbells until your back is parallel to the floor. As you bend over, you should feel a stretch in your hamstrings [2]. Keeping your back and legs straight, stand upright to return to the starting position and repeat for the prescribed number of reps.

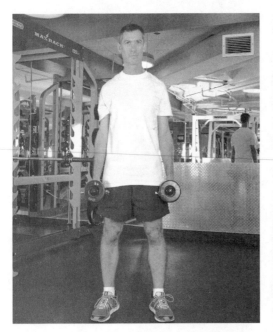

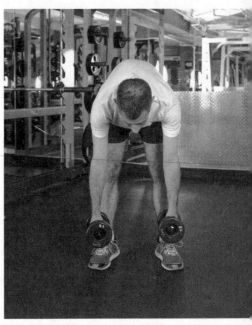

1   2

Dumbbell Row

Stand with feet shoulder-width apart with knees slightly bent and hold a dumbbell in each hand with palms facing each other. Keeping your back straight, bend over at the waist until your back is almost parallel to the floor. The dumbbells should hang directly in front of you as your arms hang perpendicular to the floor and your torso [1]. While keeping your torso stationary, use your shoulder muscles to lift the dumbbells, keeping your elbows close to your body [2]. Slowly lower the dumbbells to the starting position and repeat for the prescribed number of reps.

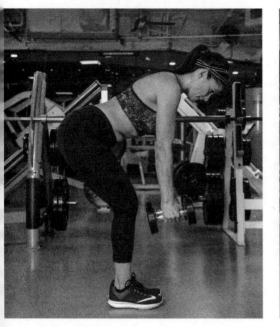

1

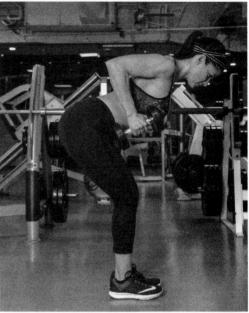

2

Dumbbell Calf Raises

Hold a dumbbell in each hand and stand with legs together, with one foot off the ground [1]. With the other foot, push against the ground with the ball of your foot to raise yourself up [2]. Slowly return to the starting position and repeat for the prescribed number of reps.

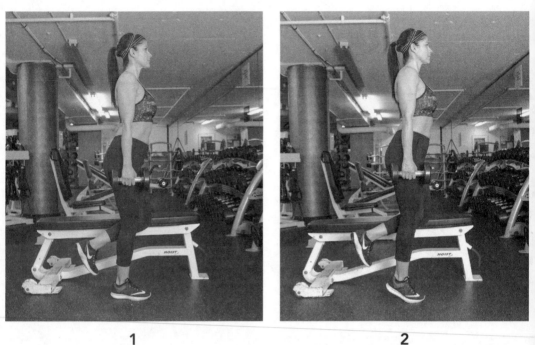

1   2

Dumbbell Biceps Curls

Stand with feet shoulder-width apart and your back straight.
Hold a dumbbell in each hand with your arms by your sides.
Keep your elbows close to your body [1]. Lift the dumbbells
by bending your elbows and rotate your hands so that your
palms face up as the dumbbells reach your shoulders [2]. Lower
the dumbbells to the starting position and repeat for the
prescribed number of reps.

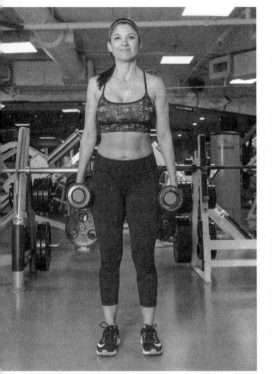
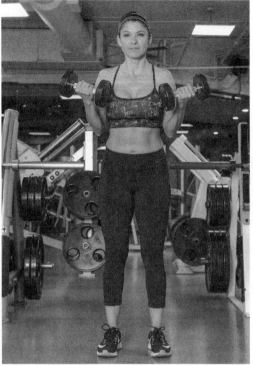

1   2

NEUROMUSCULAR STRENGTH WORKOUTS

This series of workouts makes your muscles stronger by targeting your central nervous system's ability to communicate with your muscles. The weights are very heavy, with only a few reps per set.

MACHINE WORKOUTS

Upper Body 1: Chest & Triceps

Exercise	Sets	Reps	Intensity (% 1 rep max or RPE)	Recovery
Chest Press	2–3	1–3	95%	3:00
Triceps Pressdown	2–3	1–3	95%	3:00

EXERCISE INSTRUCTIONS

Chest Press

Sit with your back straight and flat against the back pad of the machine with feet flat on the floor. Grip the handles near your chest with an overhand grip [1]. Extend your arms to push the handles forward and up to lift the weight [2]. Slowly return to the starting position to lower the weight and repeat for the prescribed number of reps.

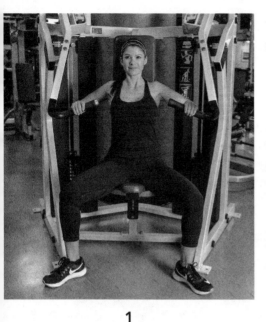
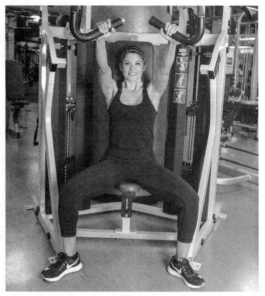

1   2

Triceps Pressdown

Attach a straight bar to a high pulley and grab the bar, using an overhand grip with your hands slightly less than shoulder-width apart. Stand with feet shoulder-width apart and your torso straight. Hold your upper arms close to your body with your elbows in to your sides and pointing down toward the floor [1]. Using your triceps, push the bar down until your arms are fully extended. Keep your upper arms stationary throughout the movement and hold them next to your torso [2]. Slowly return to the starting position to lower the weight and repeat for the prescribed number of reps.

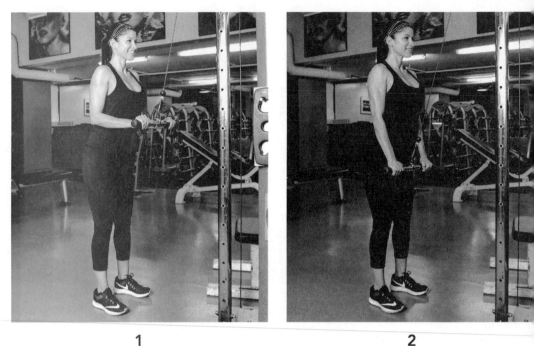

1   2

Upper Body 2: Back & Biceps

Exercise	Sets	Reps	Intensity (% 1 rep max or RPE)	Recovery
Seated Cable Row	2–3	1–3	95%	3:00
Biceps Preacher Curls	2–3	1–3	95%	3:00

EXERCISE INSTRUCTIONS

Seated Cable Row

Sit down on the machine and place your feet on the front platform with your knees slightly bent. Lean forward to grab the handles of the bar (use a V-bar that will keep your hands facing each other). Scoot back on the seat and pull the bar back with arms extended until your hips are at a 90-degree angle to your torso and your back is straight [1]. Using your back muscles, pull the handles of the bar toward your torso [2]. Slowly return to the starting position to lower the weight and repeat for the prescribed number of reps.

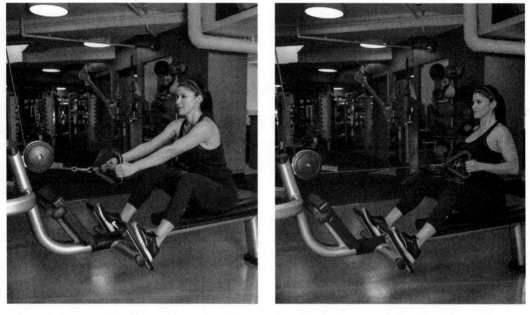

1 2

Biceps Preacher Curls

Sit on the seat of the machine and adjust the seat height so that you can comfortably extend your arms on the pad and your elbows are in line with the pivot point of the machine. Lay the back of your arms on the pad and grab the handles with an underhand grip [1]. Lift the weight by flexing your elbows, pulling your hands toward your shoulders [2]. Slowly return to the starting position to lower the weight and repeat for the prescribed number of reps.

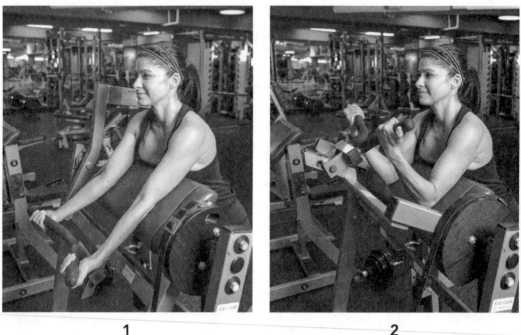

1   2

Lower Body 1: Quads & Calves

Exercise	Sets	Reps	Intensity (% 1 rep max or RPE)	Recovery
Squats (Smith machine)	2–3	1–3	95%	3:00
Calf Press	2–3	1–3	95%	3:00

EXERCISE INSTRUCTIONS

Squats (Smith machine)

Set the bar on the Smith machine to the height of your shoulders. Place any extra weight on the bar that you need to meet the prescribed intensity. With feet shoulder-width or slightly greater than shoulder-width apart, stand in front of the barbell. Place the barbell across the back of your shoulders below your neck and grab the barbell from behind with a grip slightly greater than shoulder-width. Lift the barbell from the rack so it rests on your shoulders and upper back [1]. Keeping your back straight, bend your knees and squat down until your thighs are parallel to the floor. Move your hips back as if you're going to sit in a chair [2]. Push against the floor to return to the starting position and repeat for the prescribed number of reps.

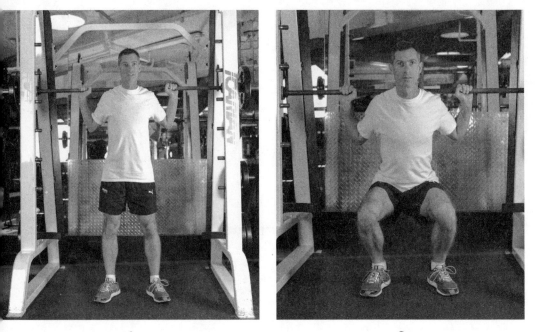

1   2

Calf Press

Sit on the seat of a seated calf press machine and place your toes and the balls of your feet on the platform in front of you with your feet shoulder-width apart, legs slightly bent, and your back against the seat cushion. Grab the side handles of the machine for support [1]. Push against the platform with the balls of your feet to lift the weight [2]. Slowly return to the starting position and repeat for the prescribed number of reps.

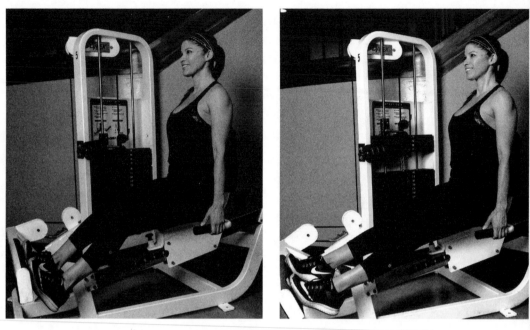

1   2

Lower Body 2: Hamstrings & Glutes

Exercise	Sets	Reps	Intensity (% 1 rep max or RPE)	Recovery
Leg Curl	2–3	1–3	95%	3:00
Hip Extension	2–3	1–3	95%	3:00

EXERCISE INSTRUCTIONS

Leg Curl

Lie facedown on the leg curl machine with your hips flat against the bench, your legs straight, and the leg pad on the back of your legs, just below your calves. Adjust the length of the lever and your position on the pad so that when you lie down, your knees are in line with the pivot point of the machine. Grab the handles of the machine for support [1]. Curl your legs up until your heels come close to your butt [2]. Slowly return to the starting position to lower the weight and repeat for the prescribed number of reps.

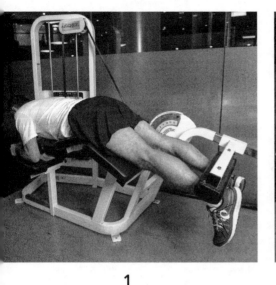
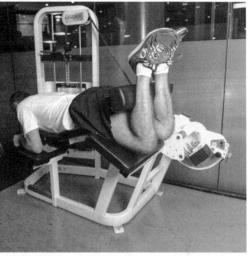

1   2

Hip Extension

Hook an ankle cuff to a low cable pulley and attach the cuff to your ankle. Stand about two feet from the machine, lean slightly forward, and grab the frame for support [1]. Squeeze your glutes and extend the cuffed leg backward, keeping the leg straight [2]. Slowly return to the starting position and repeat for the prescribed number of reps before switching to the other leg.

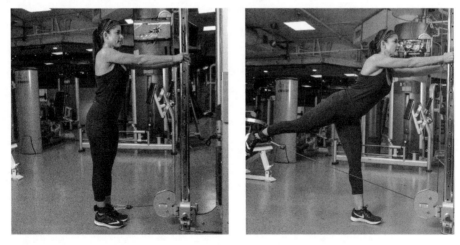

1   2

Total Body Machine Workout

Exercise	Sets	Reps	Intensity (% 1 rep max or RPE)
Leg Press	1	2–3	95%
Seated Cable Row	1	2–3	95%
Leg Curl	1	2–3	95%
Chest Press	1	2–3	95%
Hip Extension	1	2–3	95%
Shoulder Press	1	2–3	95%
Calf Press	1	2–3	95%
Biceps Preacher Curls	1	2–3	95%

Exercises alternate between lower body and upper body and progress from bigger muscles to smaller muscles. Move immediately from one exercise to the next.

EXERCISE INSTRUCTIONS

Leg Press

Sit on the leg press machine with your feet shoulder-width apart on the platform and your back flat against the back pad. Adjust the seat position so that your knees are bent at 90 degrees. Grab the side handles for support [1]. Lift the weight by pressing your feet against the platform and straightening your legs until just before your legs are completely straight [2]. Throughout the motion, keep your legs parallel to one another. Slowly return to the starting position to lower the weight and repeat for the prescribed number of reps.

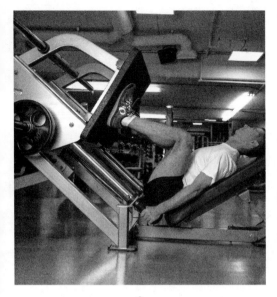

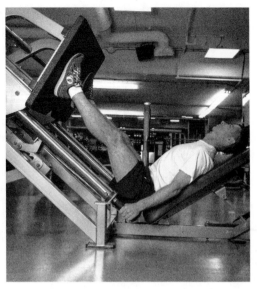

1   2

Seated Cable Row

Sit down on the machine and place your feet on the front platform with your knees slightly bent. Lean forward to grab the handles of the bar (use a V-bar that will keep your hands facing each other). Scoot back on the seat and pull the bar back with arms extended until your hips are at a 90-degree angle to your torso and your back is straight [1]. Using your back muscles, pull the handles of the bar toward your torso [2]. Slowly return to the starting position to lower the weight and repeat for the prescribed number of reps.

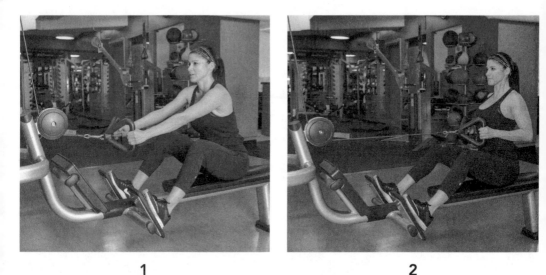

1   2

Leg Curl

Lie facedown on the leg curl machine with your hips flat against the bench, your legs straight, and the leg pad on the back of your legs, just below your calves. Adjust the length of the lever and your position on the pad so that when you lie down, your knees are in line with the pivot point of the machine. Grab the handles of the machine for support [1]. Curl your legs up until your heels come close to your butt [2]. Slowly return to the starting position to lower the weight and repeat for the prescribed number of reps.

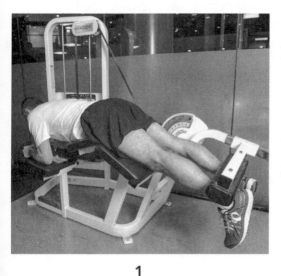
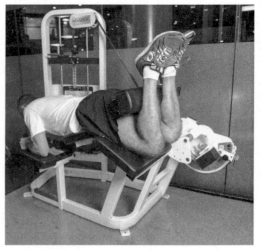

1   2

Chest Press

Sit with your back straight and flat against the back pad of the machine with feet flat on the floor. Grip the handles near your chest with an overhand grip [1]. Extend your arms to push the handles forward and up to lift the weight [2]. Slowly return to the starting position to lower the weight and repeat for the prescribed number of reps.

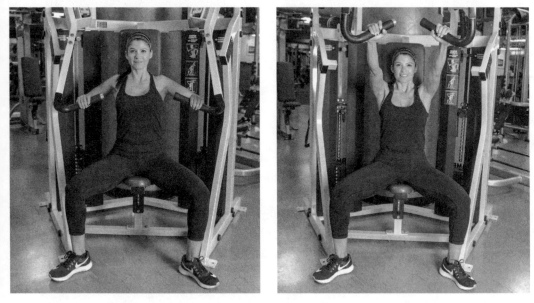

1   2

Hip Extension

Hook an ankle cuff to a low cable pulley and attach the cuff to your ankle. Stand about two feet from the machine, lean slightly forward, and grab the frame for support [1]. Squeeze your glutes and extend the cuffed leg backward, keeping the leg straight [2]. Slowly return to the starting position and repeat for the prescribed number of reps before switching to the other leg.

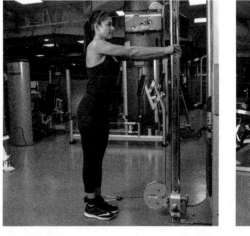

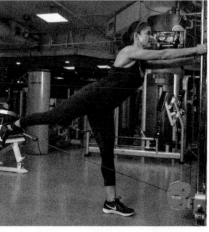

1
2

Shoulder Press

Sit down on the machine's seat with your back straight against the back pad. Adjust the seat height so that when you grab the handles, your hands are in line with your shoulders [1]. Push upward to lift the weight until your arms are fully extended [2]. Slowly return to the starting position to lower the weight and repeat for the prescribed number of reps.

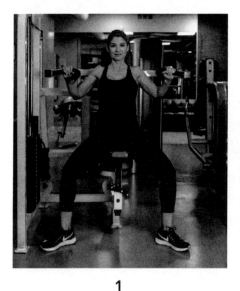

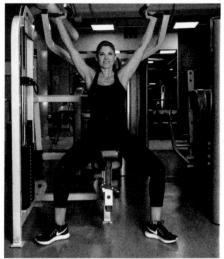

1
2

Calf Press

Sit on the seat of a seated calf press machine and place your toes and the balls of your feet on the platform in front of you with your feet shoulder-width apart, legs slightly bent, and your back against the seat cushion. Grab the side handles of the machine for support [1]. Push against the platform with the balls of your feet to lift the weight [2]. Slowly return to the starting position and repeat for the prescribed number of reps.

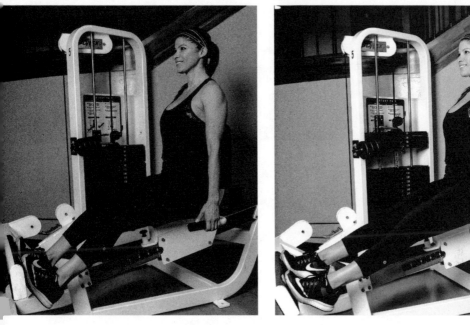

1   2

Biceps Preacher Curls

Sit on the seat of the machine and adjust the seat height so that you can comfortably extend your arms on the pad and your elbows are in line with the pivot point of the machine. Lay the back of your arms on the pad and grab the handles with an underhand grip [1]. Lift the weight by flexing your elbows, pulling your hands toward your shoulders [2]. Slowly return to the starting position to lower the weight and repeat for the prescribed number of reps.

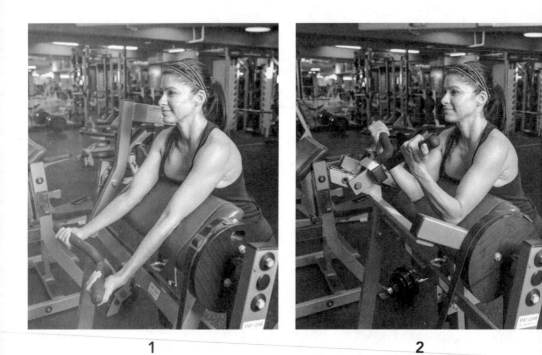

1   2

DUMBBELL WORKOUTS

Upper Body 1: Chest & Triceps

Exercise	Sets	Reps	Intensity (% 1 rep max or RPE)	Recovery
Dumbbell Chest Press	2–3	1–3	95%	3:00
Dumbbell Triceps Kickback	2–3	1–3	95%	3:00

EXERCISE INSTRUCTIONS

Dumbbell Chest Press

Grab a dumbbell in each hand with an overhand grip and lie on your back on a flat bench with your feet flat on the floor. Hold the dumbbells slightly greater than shoulder-width apart at the level of your chest with the palms of your hands facing each other and your elbows bent at 90 degrees with upper arms parallel to the floor [1]. In one curved motion, push the dumbbells upward by straightening your arms and bring the dumbbells in toward the midline of your chest while rotating your hands so that your palms face away from you as the ends of the dumbbells meet [2]. Lower the dumbbells back along the same arc to the level of your chest and repeat for the prescribed number of reps.

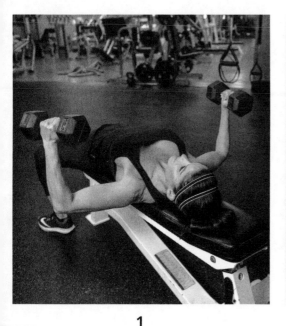

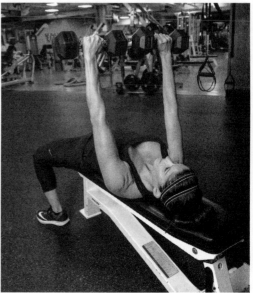

1

2

Dumbbell Triceps Kickback

Kneel on a bench with your left leg and place your left arm on the bench for support. Hold a dumbbell in your right hand with your upper arm parallel to the floor and your elbow bent at 90 degrees [1]. Extend your arm at the elbow until your arm is straight. Only your forearm should move [2]. Slowly return to the starting position and repeat for the prescribed number of reps before switching to the left arm.

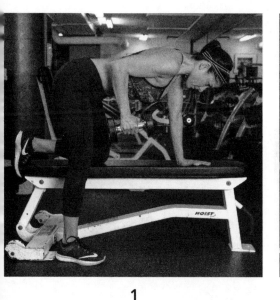
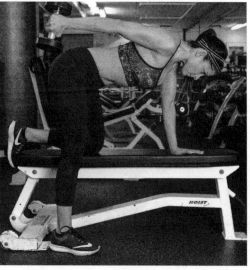

1   2

Upper Body 2: Back & Biceps

Exercise	Sets	Reps	Intensity (% 1 rep max or RPE)	Recovery
Dumbbell Reverse Flys	2–3	1–3	95%	3:00
Dumbbell Biceps Curls	2–3	1–3	95%	3:00

EXERCISE INSTRUCTIONS

Dumbbell Reverse Flys

Grab a dumbbell in each hand with an overhand grip and palms facing each other and stand with feet shoulder-width apart. Slightly bend your knees and lean forward from your hips with your back straight. Hold the dumbbells with your arms slightly bent [1]. Raise your arms out to your sides like a fly opening its wings until your elbows are slightly higher than your shoulders [2]. Lower the dumbbells to the starting position and repeat for the prescribed number of reps. You can also do this exercise on an incline bench with your torso flat against the bench [3 & 4].

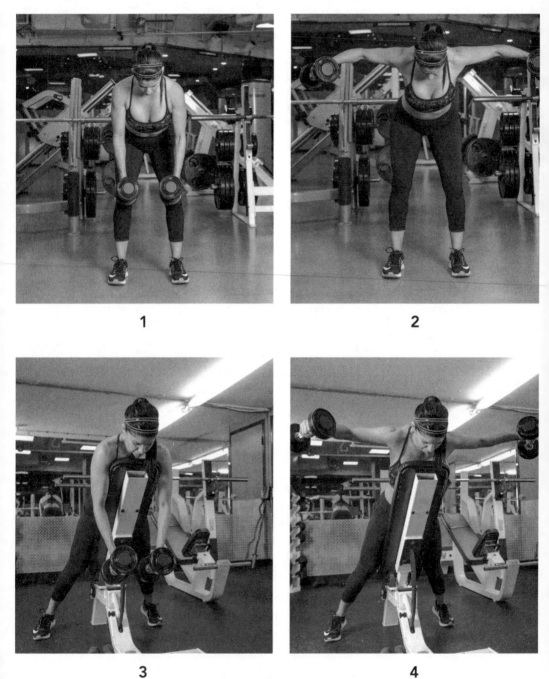

1

2

3

4

14-MINUTE METABOLIC WORKOUTS

Dumbbell Biceps Curls

Stand with feet shoulder-width apart and your back straight. Hold a dumbbell in each hand with your arms by your sides. Keep your elbows close to your body [1]. Lift the dumbbells by bending your elbows and rotate your hands so that your palms face up as the dumbbells reach your shoulders [2]. Lower the dumbbells to the starting position and repeat for the prescribed number of reps.

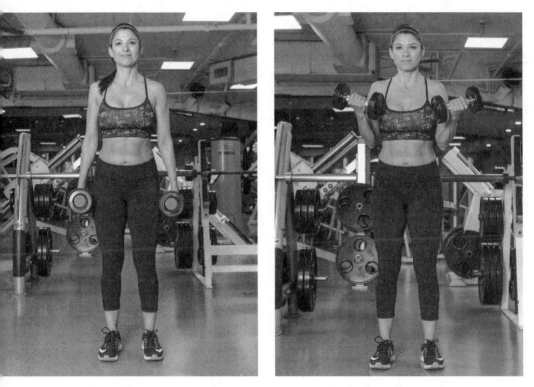

1   2

Lower Body 1: Quads & Calves

Exercise	Sets	Reps	Intensity (% 1 rep max or RPE)	Recovery
Dumbbell Squats	2–3	1–3	95%	3:00
Dumbbell Calf Raises	2–3	1–3	95%	3:00

EXERCISE INSTRUCTIONS

Dumbbell Squats

Stand with feet shoulder-width or slightly wider than shoulder-width apart with a dumbbell in each hand and arms fully extended with palms facing the side of your legs [1]. Keeping your back straight, bend your knees and squat down until your thighs are parallel to the floor. Move your hips back as if you're going to sit in a chair [2]. Push against the floor to return to the starting position and repeat for the prescribed number of reps.

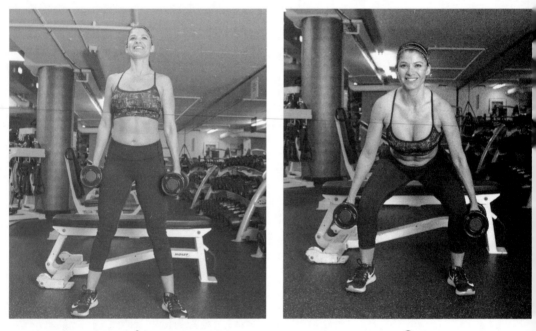

1   2

Dumbbell Calf Raises

Hold a dumbbell in each hand and stand with legs together, with one foot off the ground [1]. With the other foot, push against the ground with the ball of your foot to raise yourself up [2]. Slowly return to the starting position and repeat for the prescribed number of reps.

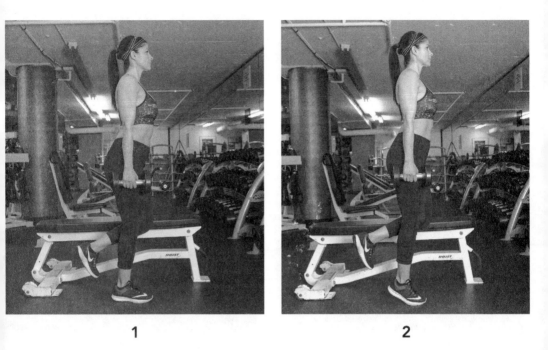

1   2

Lower Body 2: Hamstrings & Glutes

Exercise	Sets	Reps	Intensity (% 1 rep max or RPE)	Recovery
Dumbbell Deadlift	2–3	1–3	95%	3:00
Dumbbell Plié Squats	2–3	1–3	95%	3:00

EXERCISE INSTRUCTIONS

Dumbbell Deadlift

Hold a dumbbell in each hand by your sides at arm's length and stand with your feet shoulder-width apart [1]. Keeping your back and legs straight, bend over at the waist to lower the dumbbells until your back is parallel to the floor. As you bend over, you should feel a stretch in your hamstrings [2]. Keeping your back and legs straight, stand upright to return to the starting position and repeat for the prescribed number of reps.

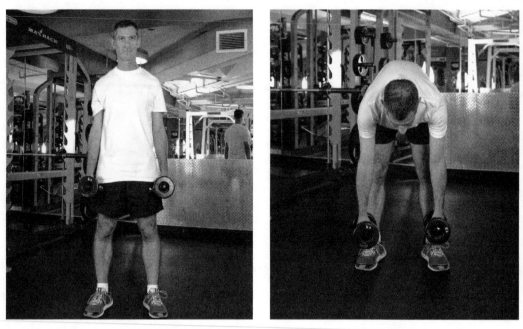

1   **2**

Dumbbell Plié Squats

Stand with feet slightly greater than shoulder-width apart and toes turned out about 45 degrees. Hold a dumbbell vertically with both hands between your legs [1]. Keeping your back straight, squat down until your thighs are parallel to the floor [2]. Push through your feet to stand up to return to the starting position and repeat for the prescribed number of reps.

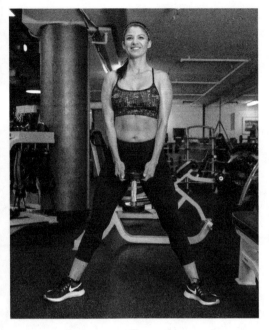
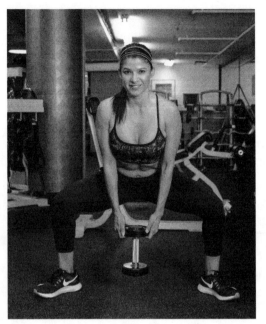

1   2

Total Body Dumbbell Workout

Exercise	Sets	Reps	Intensity (% 1 rep max or RPE)
Dumbbell Squats	1	2–3	95%
Dumbbell Chest Press	1	2–3	95%
Dumbbell Lunges	1	2–3	95%
Dumbbell Reverse Flys	1	2–3	95%
Dumbbell Deadlift	1	2–3	95%
Dumbbell Row	1	2–3	95%
Dumbbell Calf Raises	1	2–3	95%
Dumbbell Biceps Curls	1	2–3	95%

Exercises alternate between lower body and upper body and progress from bigger muscles to smaller muscles. Move immediately from one exercise to the next.

EXERCISE INSTRUCTIONS

Dumbbell Squats

Stand with feet shoulder-width or slightly wider than shoulder-width apart with a dumbbell in each hand and arms fully extended with palms facing the side of your legs [1]. Keeping your back straight, bend your knees and squat down until your thighs are parallel to the floor. Move your hips back as if you're going to sit in a chair [2]. Push against the floor to return to the starting position and repeat for the prescribed number of reps.

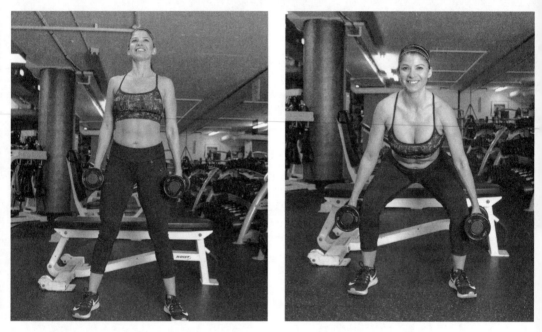

1   2

Dumbbell Chest Press

Grab a dumbbell in each hand with an overhand grip and lie on your back on a flat bench with your feet flat on the floor. Hold the dumbbells slightly greater than shoulder-width apart at the level of your chest with the palms of your hands facing each other and your elbows bent at 90 degrees with upper arms parallel to the floor [1]. In one curved motion, push the dumbbells upward by straightening your arms and bring the dumbbells in toward the midline of your chest while rotating your hands so that your palms face away from you as the ends of the dumbbells meet [2]. Lower the dumbbells back along the same arc to the level of your chest and repeat for the prescribed number of reps.

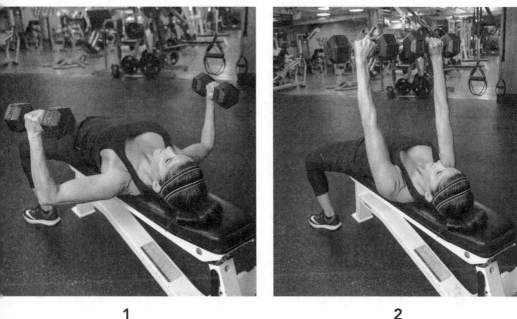

1   2

Dumbbell Lunges

Stand with your torso upright, holding a dumbbell in each hand by your sides [1]. Step forward about two feet with your right leg and lower yourself down into the lunge while keeping your torso upright. Keep your right knee above your toes as you lunge forward and keep your right shin perpendicular to the ground [2]. Push yourself back up and lunge forward with your left leg. Repeat for the prescribed number of reps.

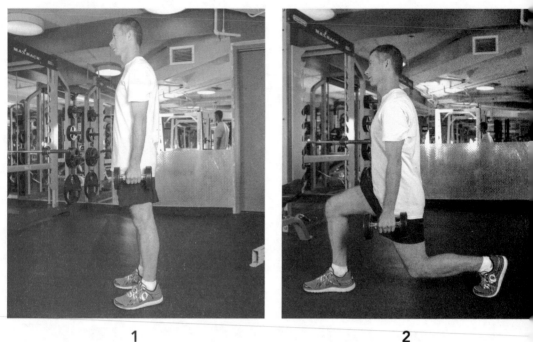

1   2

Dumbbell Reverse Flys

Grab a dumbbell in each hand with an overhand grip and palms facing each other and stand with feet shoulder-width apart. Slightly bend your knees and lean forward from your hips with your back straight. Hold the dumbbells with your arms slightly bent [1]. Raise your arms out to your sides like a fly opening its wings until your elbows are slightly higher than your shoulders [2]. Lower the dumbbells to the starting position and repeat for the prescribed number of reps. You can also do this exercise on an incline bench with your torso flat against the bench [3 & 4].

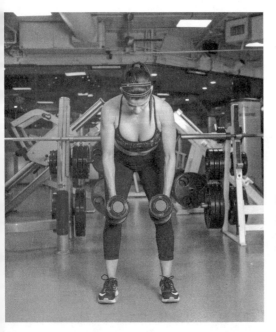

1

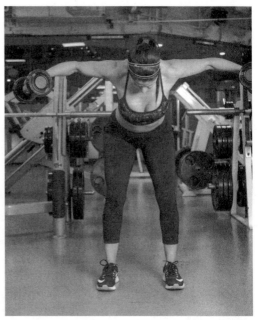

2

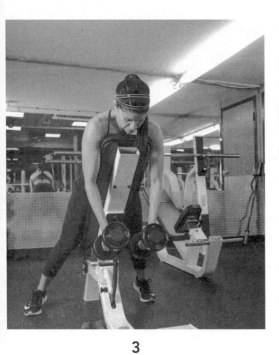

3

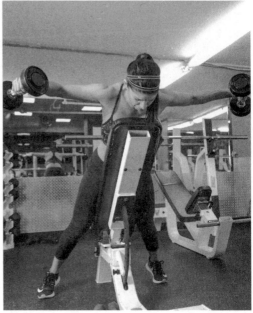

4

Dumbbell Deadlift

Hold a dumbbell in each hand by your sides at arm's length and stand with your feet shoulder-width apart [1]. Keeping your back and legs straight, bend over at the waist to lower the dumbbells until your back is parallel to the floor. As you bend over, you should feel a stretch in your hamstrings [2]. Keeping your back and legs straight, stand upright to return to the starting position and repeat for the prescribed number of reps.

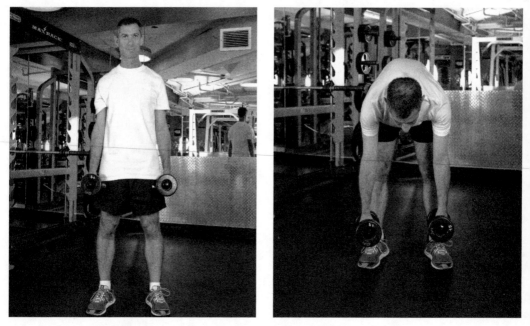

1   2

Dumbbell Row

Stand with feet shoulder-width apart with knees slightly bent and hold a dumbbell in each hand with palms facing each other. Keeping your back straight, bend over at the waist until your back is almost parallel to the floor. The dumbbells should hang directly in front of you as your arms hang perpendicular to the floor and your torso [1]. While keeping your torso stationary, use your shoulder muscles to lift the dumbbells, keeping your elbows close to your body [2]. Slowly lower the dumbbells to the starting position and repeat for the prescribed number of reps.

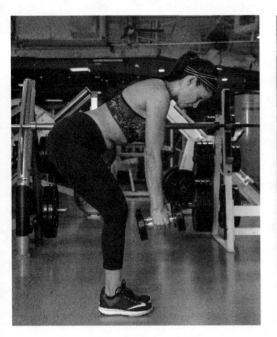

1

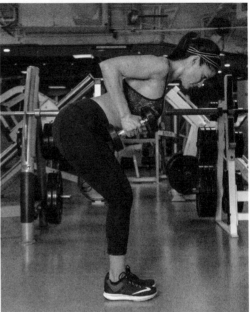

2

Dumbbell Calf Raises

Hold a dumbbell in each hand and stand with legs together, with one foot off the ground [1]. With the other foot, push against the ground with the ball of your foot to raise yourself up [2]. Slowly return to the starting position and repeat for the prescribed number of reps.

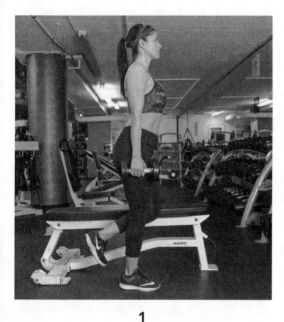
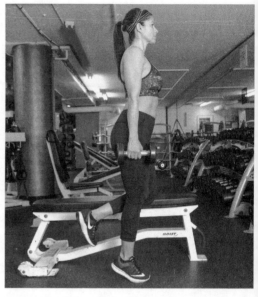

1

2

Dumbbell Biceps Curls

Stand with feet shoulder-width apart and your back straight.
Hold a dumbbell in each hand with your arms by your sides.
Keep your elbows close to your body [1]. Lift the dumbbells
by bending your elbows and rotate your hands so that your
palms face up as the dumbbells reach your shoulders [2]. Lower
the dumbbells to the starting position and repeat for the
prescribed number of reps.

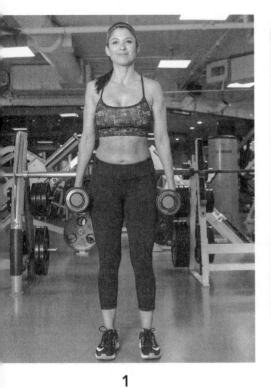
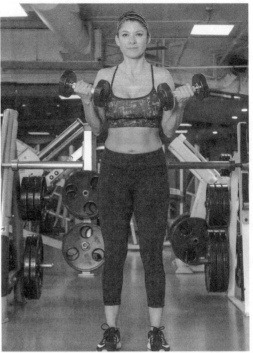

1   2

MUSCULAR POWER WORKOUTS

This series of workouts improves the speed at which your muscles generate force. For all exercises, move the weight as quickly as you can without sacrificing form.

MACHINE WORKOUTS

Upper Body 1: Back & Biceps

Exercise	Sets	Reps	Intensity (% 1 rep max or RPE)	Recovery
Chin-Ups	2	10	30–50%	3:00
Seated Cable Row	2	10	30–50%	3:00
Biceps Preacher Curls	2	10	30–50%	3:00

Move the weight fast (but still under control) to focus on the speed component of muscular power.

EXERCISE INSTRUCTIONS

Chin-Ups

Stand on the platform of a weight-assisted chin-up machine. Grab the handles of the machine above your head with an underhand grip [1]. Pull yourself up until your chin reaches the height of your hands [2]. Lower yourself down to the starting position and repeat for the prescribed number of reps.

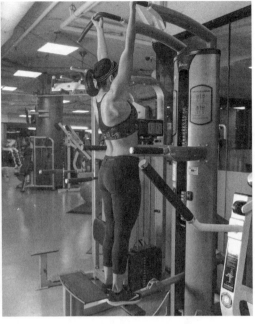

1

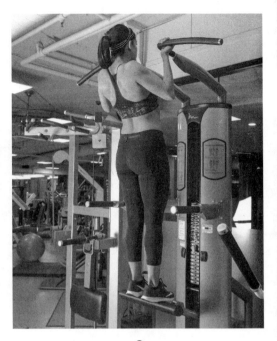

2

Seated Cable Row

Sit down on the machine and place your feet on the front platform with your knees slightly bent. Lean forward to grab the handles of the bar (use a V-bar that will keep your hands facing each other). Scoot back on the seat and pull the bar back with arms extended until your hips are at a 90-degree angle to your torso and your back is straight [1]. Using your back muscles, pull the handles of the bar toward your torso [2]. Slowly return to the starting position to lower the weight and repeat for the prescribed number of reps.

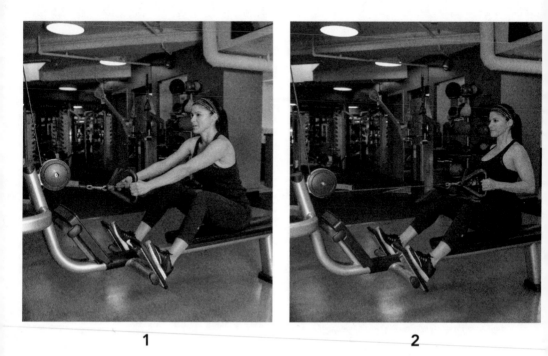

1   2

Biceps Preacher Curls

Sit on the seat of the machine and adjust the seat height so that you can comfortably extend your arms on the pad and your elbows are in line with the pivot point of the machine. Lay the back of your arms on the pad and grab the handles with an underhand grip [1]. Lift the weight by flexing your elbows, pulling your hands toward your shoulders [2]. Slowly return to the starting position to lower the weight and repeat for the prescribed number of reps.

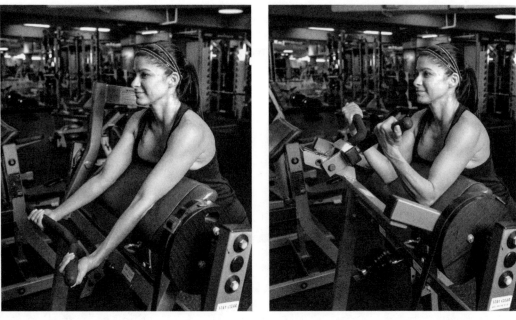

1   2

Upper Body 2: Chest, Shoulders, & Triceps

Exercise	Sets	Reps	Intensity (% 1 rep max or RPE)	Recovery
Chest Press	2	10	30–50%	3:00
Shoulder Press	2	10	30–50%	3:00
Triceps Pressdown	2	10	30–50%	3:00

Move the weight fast (but still under control) to focus on the speed component of muscular power.

EXERCISE INSTRUCTIONS

Chest Press

Sit with your back straight and flat against the back pad of the machine with feet flat on the floor. Grip the handles near your chest with an overhand grip [1]. Extend your arms to push the handles forward and up to lift the weight [2]. Slowly return to the starting position to lower the weight and repeat for the prescribed number of reps.

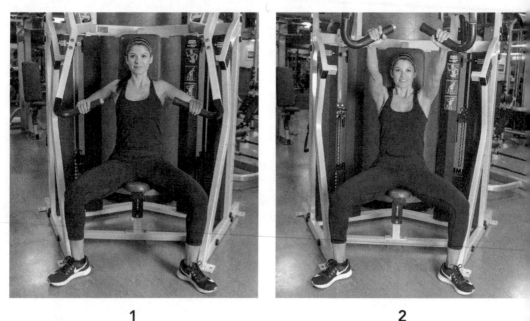

1   2

Shoulder Press

Sit down on the machine's seat with your back straight against the back pad. Adjust the seat height so that when you grab the handles, your hands are in line with your shoulders [1]. Push upward to lift the weight until your arms are fully extended [2]. Slowly return to the starting position to lower the weight and repeat for the prescribed number of reps.

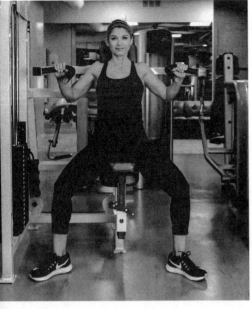
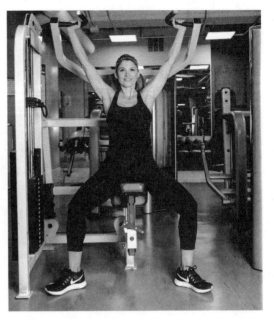

1   2

Triceps Pressdown

Attach a straight bar to a high pulley and grab the bar, using an overhand grip with your hands slightly less than shoulder-width apart. Stand with feet shoulder-width apart and your torso straight. Hold your upper arms close to your body with your elbows in to your sides and pointing down toward the floor [1]. Using your triceps, push the bar down until your arms are fully extended. Keep your upper arms stationary throughout the movement and hold them next to your torso [2]. Slowly return to the starting position to lower the weight and repeat for the prescribed number of reps.

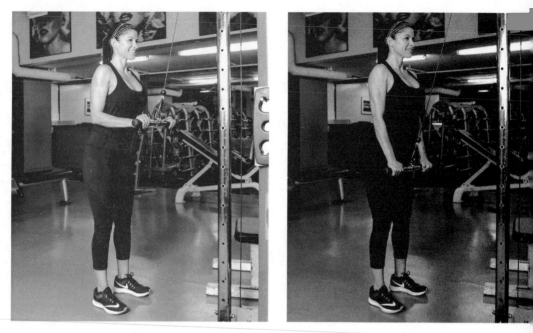

1   2

Lower Body 1: Quads & Calves

Exercise	Sets	Reps	Intensity (% 1 rep max or RPE)	Recovery
Squats (Smith machine)	2	10	30–50%	3:00
Calf Press	2	10	30–50%	3:00
Leg Press	2	10	30–50%	3:00

Move the weight fast (but still under control) to focus on the speed component of muscular power.

EXERCISE INSTRUCTIONS

Squats (Smith machine)

Set the bar on the Smith machine to the height of your shoulders. Place any extra weight on the bar that you need to meet the prescribed intensity. With feet shoulder-width or slightly greater than shoulder-width apart, stand in front of the barbell. Place the barbell across the back of your shoulders below your neck and grab the barbell from behind with a grip slightly greater than shoulder-width. Lift the barbell from the rack so it rests on your shoulders and upper back [1]. Keeping your back straight, bend your knees and squat down until your thighs are parallel to the floor. Move your hips back as if you're going to sit in a chair [2]. Push against the floor to return to the starting position and repeat for the prescribed number of reps.

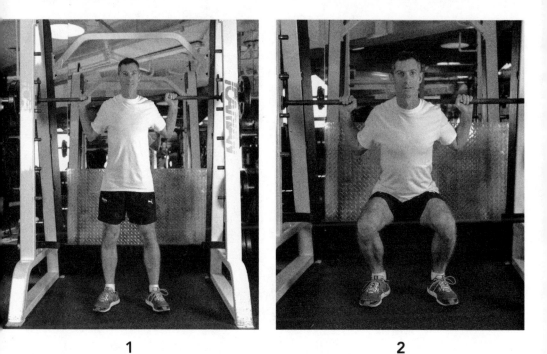

1   2

Calf Press

Sit on the seat of a seated calf press machine and place your toes and the balls of your feet on the platform in front of you with your feet shoulder-width apart, legs slightly bent, and your back against the seat cushion. Grab the side handles of the machine for support [1]. Push against the platform with the balls of your feet to lift the weight [2]. Slowly return to the starting position and repeat for the prescribed number of reps.

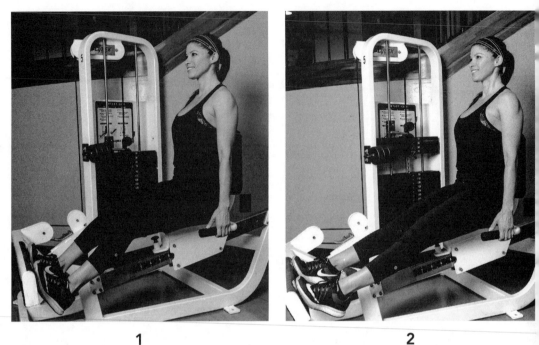

1 2

Leg Press

Sit on the leg press machine with your feet shoulder-width apart on the platform and your back flat against the back pad. Adjust the seat position so that your knees are bent at 90 degrees. Grab the side handles for support [1]. Lift the weight by pressing your feet against the platform and straightening your legs until just before your legs are completely straight [2]. Throughout the motion, keep your legs parallel to one another. Slowly return to the starting position to lower the weight and repeat for the prescribed number of reps.

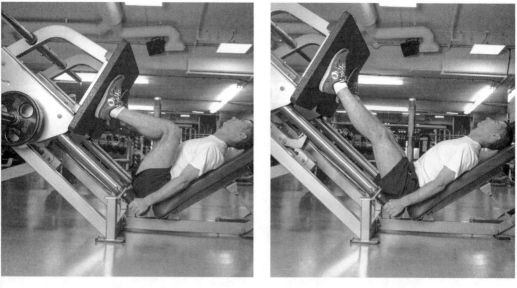

| 1 | 2 |

Lower Body 2: Hamstrings, Glutes, & Inner Thighs

Exercise	Sets	Reps	Intensity (% 1 rep max or RPE)	Recovery
Leg Curl	2	10	30–50%	3:00
Hip Extension	2	10	30–50%	3:00
Low-Cable Deadlift	2	10	30–50%	3:00

Move the weight fast (but still under control) to focus on the speed component of muscular power.

EXERCISE INSTRUCTIONS

Leg Curl

Lie facedown on the leg curl machine with your hips flat against the bench, your legs straight, and the leg pad on the back of your legs, just below your calves. Adjust the length of the lever and your position on the pad so that when you lie down, your knees are in line with the pivot point of the machine. Grab the handles of the machine for support [1]. Curl your legs up until your heels come close to your butt [2]. Slowly return to the starting position to lower the weight and repeat for the prescribed number of reps.

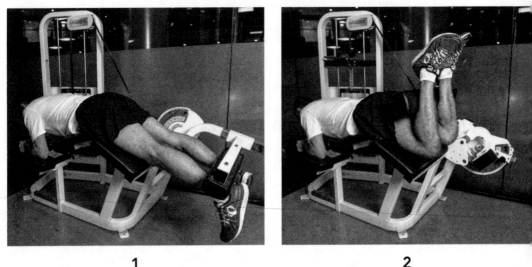

1   2

Hip Extension

Hook an ankle cuff to a low cable pulley and attach the cuff to your ankle. Stand about two feet from the machine, lean slightly forward, and grab the frame for support [1]. Squeeze your glutes and extend the cuffed leg backward, keeping the leg straight [2]. Slowly return to the starting position and repeat for the prescribed number of reps before switching to the other leg.

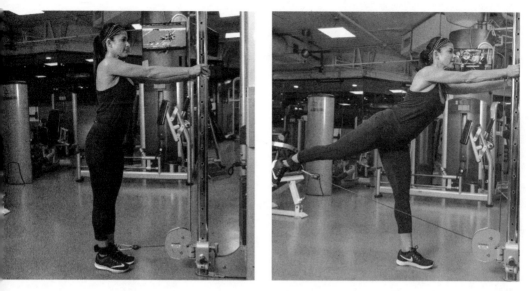

1   2

Low-Cable Deadlift

Attach a straight bar to the cable machine and set it to the lowest setting. Grab the bar with an overhand, shoulder-width grip and step back about two steps. Stand with your feet shoulder-width apart, legs straight or slightly bent, and bend over from your waist with your back straight [1]. Lift the bar by raising your torso to stand up straight, keeping your legs and back straight [2]. Slowly lower the bar to the starting position and repeat for the prescribed number of reps.

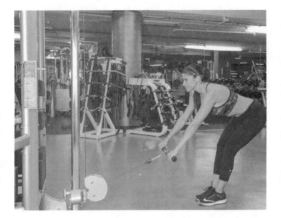

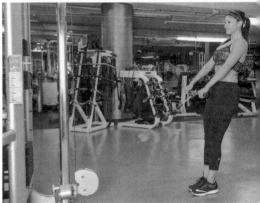

1   2

Total Body Machine Workout

Exercise	Sets	Reps	Intensity (% 1 rep max or RPE)
Leg Press	1	10	30–50%
Seated Cable Row	1	10	30–50%
Leg Curl	1	10	30–50%
Chest Press	1	10	30–50%
Hip Extension	1	10	30–50%
Shoulder Press	1	10	30–50%
Calf Press	1	10	30–50%
Biceps Preacher Curls	1	10	30–50%

Exercises alternate between lower body and upper body and progress from bigger muscles to smaller muscles. Move immediately from one exercise to the next. Move the weight fast (but still under control) to focus on the speed component of muscular power.

EXERCISE INSTRUCTIONS

Leg Press

Sit on the leg press machine with your feet shoulder-width apart on the platform and your back flat against the back pad. Adjust the seat position so that your knees are bent at 90 degrees. Grab the side handles for support [1]. Lift the weight by pressing your feet against the platform and straightening your legs until just before your legs are completely straight [2]. Throughout the motion, keep your legs parallel to one another. Slowly return to the starting position to lower the weight and repeat for the prescribed number of reps.

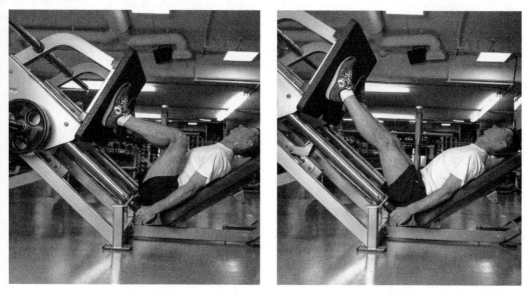

1   2

Seated Cable Row

Sit down on the machine and place your feet on the front platform with your knees slightly bent. Lean forward to grab the handles of the bar (use a V-bar that will keep your hands facing each other). Scoot back on the seat and pull the bar back with arms extended until your hips are at a 90-degree angle to your torso and your back is straight [1]. Using your back muscles, pull the handles of the bar toward your torso [2]. Slowly return to the starting position to lower the weight and repeat for the prescribed number of reps.

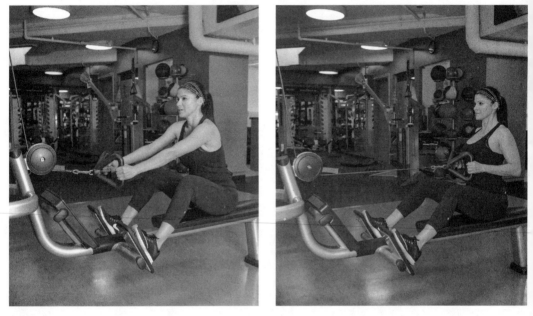

1   2

Leg Curl

Lie facedown on the leg curl machine with your hips flat against the bench, your legs straight, and the leg pad on the back of your legs, just below your calves. Adjust the length of the lever and your position on the pad so that when you lie down, your knees are in line with the pivot point of the machine. Grab the handles of the machine for support [1]. Curl your legs up until your heels come close to your butt [2]. Slowly return to the starting position to lower the weight and repeat for the prescribed number of reps.

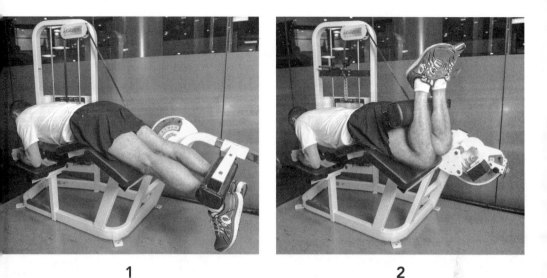

1

2

Chest Press

Sit with your back straight and flat against the back pad of the machine with feet flat on the floor. Grip the handles near your chest with an overhand grip [1]. Extend your arms to push the handles forward and up to lift the weight [2]. Slowly return to the starting position to lower the weight and repeat for the prescribed number of reps.

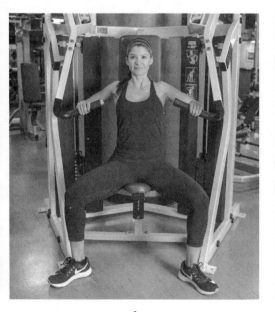

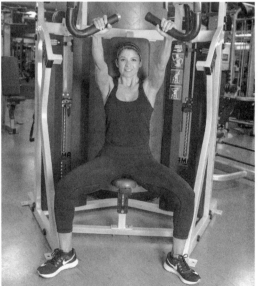

1

2

Hip Extension

Hook an ankle cuff to a low cable pulley and attach the cuff to your ankle. Stand about two feet from the machine, lean slightly forward, and grab the frame for support [1]. Squeeze your glutes and extend the cuffed leg backward, keeping the leg straight [2]. Slowly return to the starting position and repeat for the prescribed number of reps before switching to the other leg.

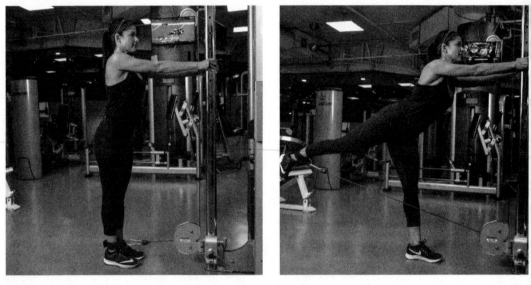

1   2

Shoulder Press

Sit down on the machine's seat with your back straight against the back pad. Adjust the seat height so that when you grab the handles, your hands are in line with your shoulders [1]. Push upward to lift the weight until your arms are fully extended [2]. Slowly return to the starting position to lower the weight and repeat for the prescribed number of reps.

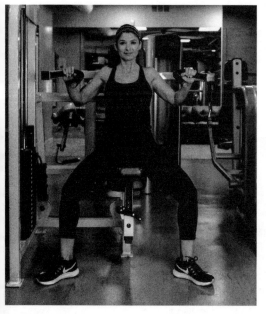
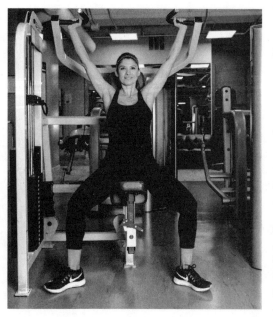

1 2

Calf Press

Sit on the seat of a seated calf press machine and place your toes and the balls of your feet on the platform in front of you with your feet shoulder-width apart, legs slightly bent, and your back against the seat cushion. Grab the side handles of the machine for support [1]. Push against the platform with the balls of your feet to lift the weight [2]. Slowly return to the starting position and repeat for the prescribed number of reps.

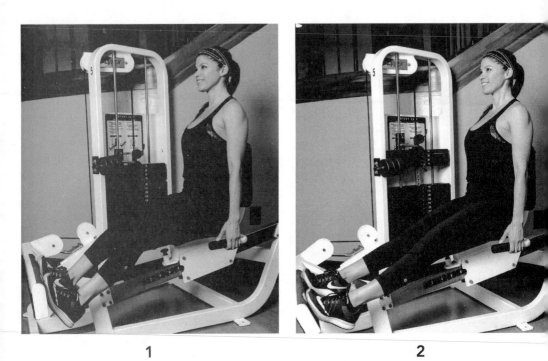

1

2

Biceps Preacher Curls

Sit on the seat of the machine and adjust the seat height so that you can comfortably extend your arms on the pad and your elbows are in line with the pivot point of the machine. Lay the back of your arms on the pad and grab the handles with an underhand grip [1]. Lift the weight by flexing your elbows, pulling your hands toward your shoulders [2]. Slowly return to the starting position to lower the weight and repeat for the prescribed number of reps.

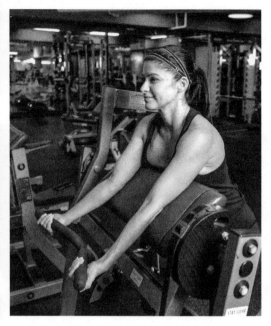
1

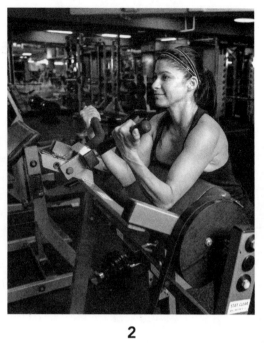
2

PLYOMETRIC WORKOUTS

Plyometric Power Workout

Exercise	Reps	Sets	Recovery
Single-Leg Hops	10 each leg	2	2:00
Stair Hops	10 each leg	2	2:00
Alternate-Leg Bound	10 each leg	2	2:00
Tuck Jumps	10	2	2:00
Depth Jumps	10	2	2:00
Platform Jumps	10	2	2:00

Do these plyometric exercises on a soft surface with good footing, like grass, artificial turf, or a yoga mat. Spend as little time on the ground as possible between hops, bounds, and jumps. Think of your legs like springs and focus on exploding off the ground.

EXERCISE INSTRUCTIONS

Single-Leg Hops

Stand with feet together. Pick your left leg up off the ground [1]. Keeping your right leg straight, hop up and down on the ball of your foot [2]. Repeat for the prescribed number of reps before switching to the left leg.

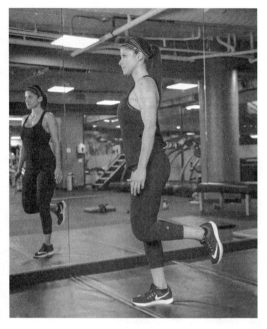
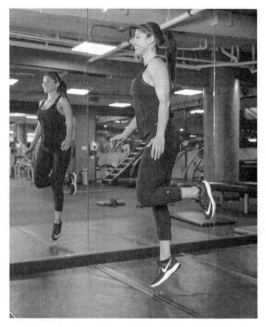

1   **2**

Stair Hops

Stand on your right leg at the bottom of a flight of stairs [1]. With your leg straight, hop up the stairs like a pogo stick, pushing off the ball of your foot [2]. Repeat for the prescribed number of reps before switching to the left leg.

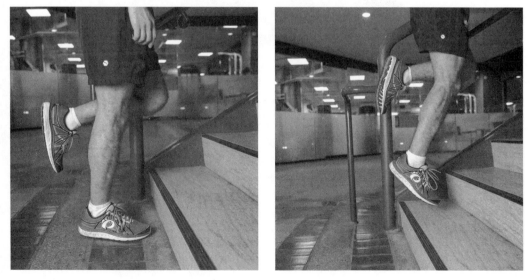

1   **2**

Alternate-Leg Bound

Leap forward off your left leg. As soon as you land on your right foot, push off the ground to leap forward off your right leg. Swing your arms from your shoulders as you would when you run, exaggerating the range of motion. Continue bounding from one leg to the other for the prescribed number of reps.

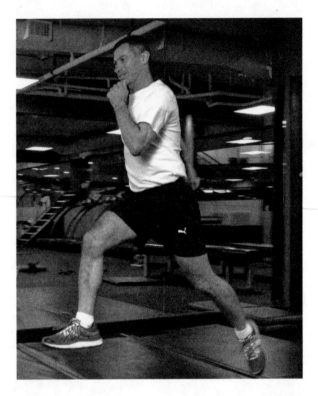

Tuck Jumps

Stand with feet shoulder-width apart. Hold your arms out in front of you over your legs [1]. Bend your knees and rapidly squat down into a quarter to half squat [2] and immediately jump up as high as you can as you lift your knees, tapping them with your hands [3]. Land with soft knees, lowering yourself back into the quarter- to half-squat position in one smooth motion, and immediately jump up again. Repeat for the prescribed number of reps.

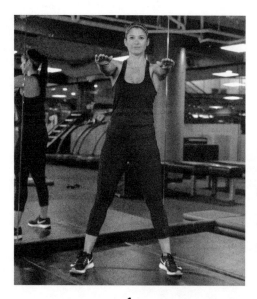

1

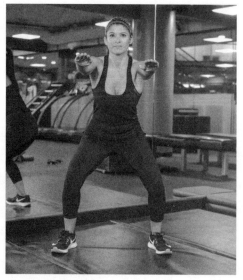

2

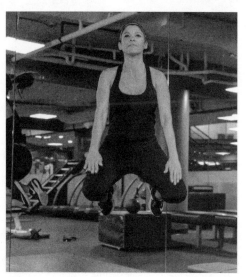

3

Depth Jumps

Stand on a firm platform about two feet tall with your legs
shoulder-width apart [1]. Jump onto the ground and land in a squat
position with your thighs parallel to the ground and your knees in
line with your toes [2]. From this squat position, jump straight up as
high as possible [3]. Repeat for the prescribed number of reps.

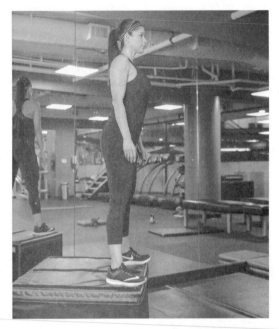

1

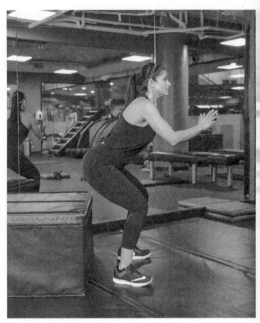

2

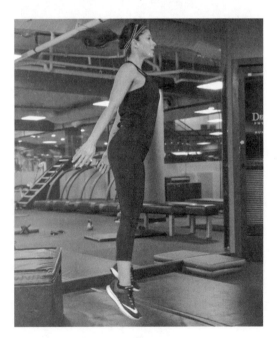

3

14-MINUTE METABOLIC WORKOUTS

Platform Jumps

Stand in front of a firm platform about two feet high in a squat position with your feet shoulder-width apart and knees bent [1]. Jump with two feet onto the platform [2]. As soon as you land, jump into the air and back down to the ground on the other side of the platform [3]. To make the exercise more challenging, jump with one foot at a time. Repeat for the prescribed number of reps.

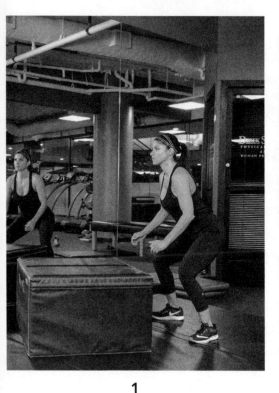

1

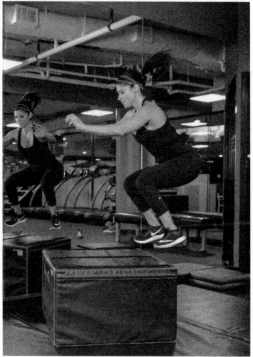

2

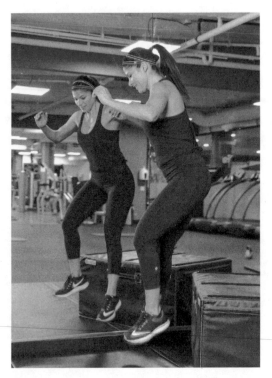

3

Power Circuit

Exercise	Reps
Squat Jumps	15–20
Dumbbell Single-Arm Swings	15–20 each arm
Split-Jump Lunges	15–20
Renegades	15–20
Single-Leg Hops	15–20 each leg
Medicine Ball Toss	15–20
Tuck Jumps	15–20
Dumbbell Chest Press	15–20

This power circuit alternates a lower-body power exercise with an upper-body power exercise. Do each exercise fast and go immediately from one exercise to the next. Do the circuit once or twice with 5 minutes rest between sets.

EXERCISE INSTRUCTIONS

Squat Jumps

Begin in a squat position with thighs parallel to the ground and hands on your hips [1]. Jump straight up as high as you can [2]. Land with soft knees, lowering yourself back into the squat position in one smooth motion, and immediately jump up again. Repeat for the prescribed number of reps.

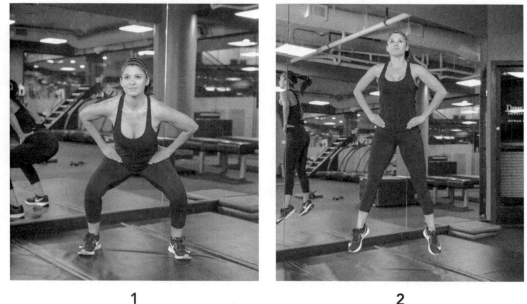

1   2

Dumbbell Single-Arm Swings

Stand up straight, with feet slightly wider than shoulder-width apart. Grab the dumbbell with your right hand, keeping your palm facedown and arm in front of your body. Bend your knees slightly and drive your hips back as you swing the dumbbell between your legs [1]. Explosively drive your hips forward while swinging the dumbbell upward until your arm is parallel to the ground [2]. Swing the dumbbell back down to the starting position and quickly transfer it to your left hand as it passes through your legs. Repeat the swing with your left arm and continue alternating hands for the prescribed number of reps.

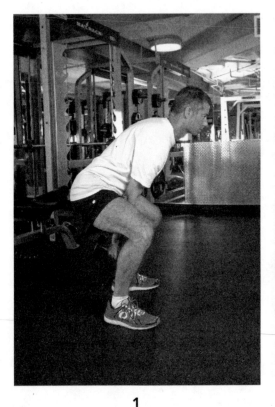

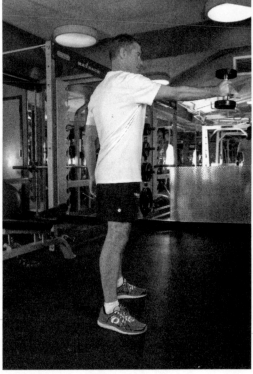

1

2

Split-Jump Lunges

Stand with your feet shoulder-width apart. Step forward about two feet with your right leg and lower yourself down into the lunge while keeping your torso upright. Keep your right knee above your toes as you lunge forward and keep your right shin perpendicular to the ground [1]. From this lunge position, jump up into the air with both feet while switching your leg position in midair [2] and land with your left leg forward [3]. Repeat for the prescribed number of reps.

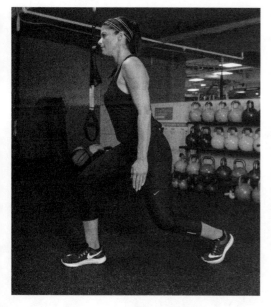

1

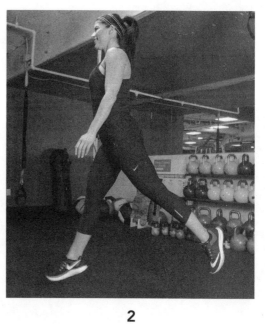

2

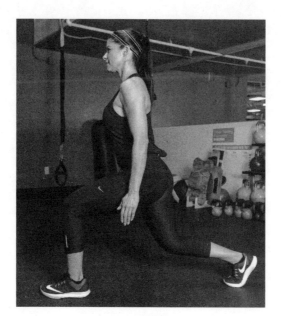

3

Renegades

Stand with your legs shoulder-width apart, bend at the waist, and hold a dumbbell in each hand with arms hanging down in front of you and palms facing each other [1]. Bend your right elbow to quickly pull the dumbbell to your chest [2]. Lower that dumbbell and quickly pull the dumbbell in your left hand to your chest [3]. Keep alternating arms and repeat for the prescribed number of reps.

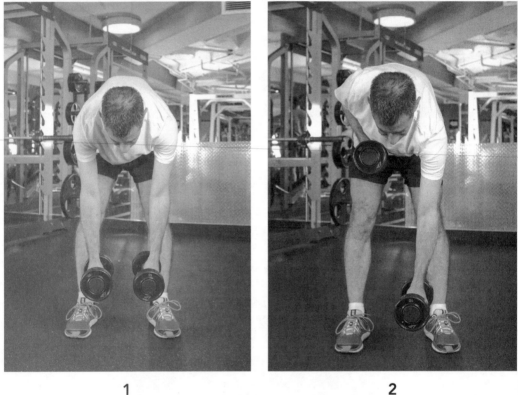

1   2

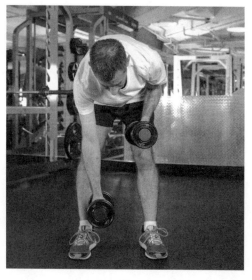

3

Single-Leg Hops

Stand with feet together. Pick your left leg up off the ground [1]. Keeping your right leg straight, hop up and down on the ball of your foot [2]. Repeat for the prescribed number of reps before switching to the left leg.

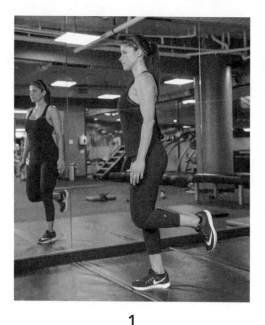

1

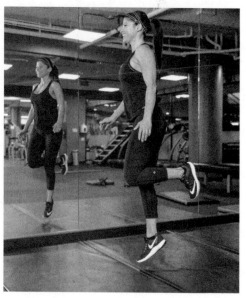

2

Medicine Ball Toss

Stand with feet shoulder-width apart. With your knees slightly bent and core tight, throw an 8- to 10-pound medicine ball with two hands from your chest straight up into the air like a volleyball pass [1–2]. Catch the medicine ball with outstretched arms, drawing your arms into your chest in one smooth movement and quickly throw it back up again. Repeat for the prescribed number of reps.

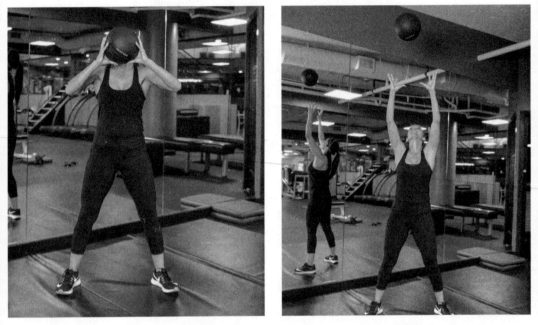

1   2

Tuck Jumps

Stand with feet shoulder-width apart. Hold your arms out in front of you over your legs [1]. Bend your knees and rapidly squat down into a quarter to half squat [2] and immediately jump up as high as you can as you lift your knees, tapping them with your hands [3]. Land with soft knees, lowering yourself back into the quarter- to half-squat position in one smooth motion, and immediately jump up again. Repeat for the prescribed number of reps.

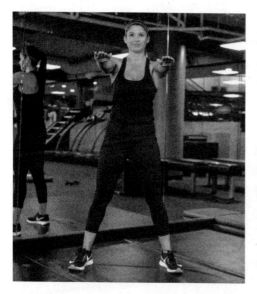

1

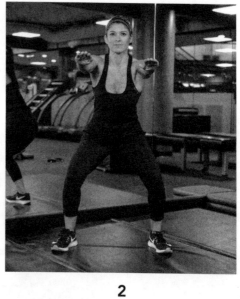

2

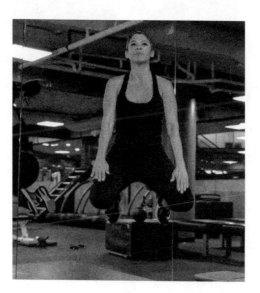

3

Dumbbell Chest Press

Grab a dumbbell in each hand with an overhand grip and lie on your back on a flat bench with your feet flat on the floor. Hold the dumbbells slightly greater than shoulder-width apart at the level of your chest with the palms of your hands facing each other and your elbows bent at 90 degrees with upper arms parallel to the floor [1]. In one curved motion, quickly push the dumbbells upward by straightening your arms and bring the dumbbells in toward the midline of your chest while rotating your hands so that your palms face away from you as the ends of the dumbbells meet [2]. Quickly lower the dumbbells back along the same arc to the level of your chest and repeat for the prescribed number of reps.

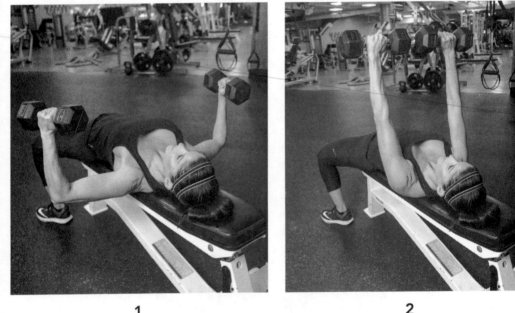

1   2

CHAPTER 5

FLEXIBILITY WORKOUTS

I used to be a big believer in stretching. It was how my middle school and high school classmates and I started physical education class every day. It's what my track coaches had me and my teammates do every day at the start of track practice. Bend down, touch your toes, cross one leg over the other, and bend down and touch your toes again. It became my daily pre-run ritual.

If you've ever run with a dog or watched a horse race, you've probably noticed something interesting—other animals don't stretch before or after they exercise. When a lion in the wild sees his dinner running by, he doesn't pause to stretch his hamstrings before chasing it. Other animals stretch only occasionally, like when waking from a nap, perhaps because it feels good. The lion may be on to something because, truth is, there is little scientific evidence for much of what is commonly accepted about stretching.

But we're not lions.

Although it's true that stretching has limitations beyond what your high school gym teacher taught you—it doesn't improve your exercise or sport performance, reduce your risk of injuries, or reduce muscle soreness after your workouts—it does improve flexibility, which is important for humans. Indeed, flexibility—the range of motion around a joint—is one of the five components of physical fitness. Other animals live with a limited amount of flexibility. They don't need to bend down a few feet to tie their shoes or reach above their heads to change a light bulb or turn around while in the driver's seat to scold their twin children in the back of the car because they're fighting with each other, like my mother used to do.

Despite the stretching that your gym teacher made your class do before all those wind sprints along the gym floor, stretching is actually more effective if you do it apart from your other workouts. So, instead of stretching before or even after you do the workouts in the previous chapters, use the flexibility exercises in this chapter as stand-alone workouts. Your hamstrings will thank you.

STATIC STRETCHING

Static stretching is the most common method of stretching, during which you move to the end of your limb's range of motion and hold the position.

Static Stretching Workout

Exercise	Duration
Static Glute Stretch	:15 each leg
Static Hamstrings Stretch	:15 each leg
Static Quadriceps Stretch	:15 each leg
Static Adductor Stretch	:15 each leg
Static Hip Flexor Stretch	:15 each leg
Static Calf Stretch	:15 each leg
Static Shoulder Stretch	:15 each arm
Static Triceps Stretch	:15 each arm

After you have completed this workout a few times, repeat each stretch a second time for a total workout time of 8 minutes.

EXERCISE INSTRUCTIONS

Static Glute Stretch

Sit with your legs out in front of you. Bend your right leg and cross it over your left leg, placing your right foot on the ground to the left side of your left knee [1]. Turn your shoulders so that you're facing to the right. Press your left arm against your right knee to help you twist to the side. Put your right arm on the ground for support [2]. Feel the stretch in your right glutes and along the length of your spine. Hold the stretch for the prescribed duration and repeat with your left leg.

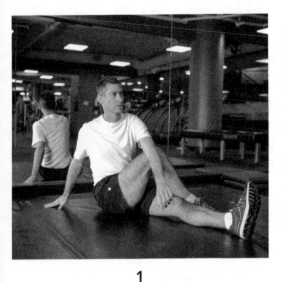
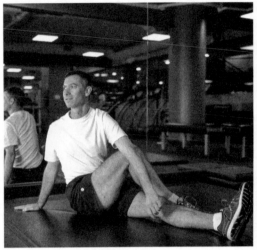

1 **2**

Static Hamstrings Stretch

Sit on the ground with both legs straight out in front of you. Bend your left leg and place the sole of your left foot along the inside of your right leg [1]. Bend forward to reach your right toes [2]. Feel the stretch in the hamstrings of your right leg. Hold the stretch for the prescribed duration and repeat with your left leg.

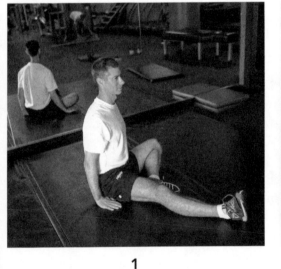
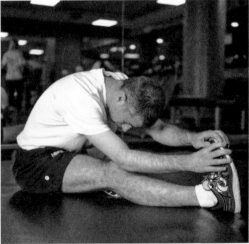

1 **2**

Static Quadriceps Stretch

Standing next to a wall or chair for balance, bend your left knee and bring your left foot toward your butt [1]. Grab your left foot with your left hand. Keep your back straight and don't bend forward at the hips [2]. Feel the stretch in your left quadriceps. Hold the stretch for the prescribed duration and repeat with your right leg.

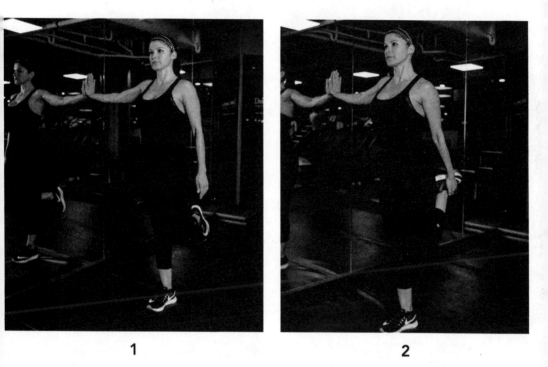

1   2

Static Adductor Stretch

Standing with your feet approximately two shoulder-widths apart, bend your left leg and lower your body toward your left side, keeping your back straight. Keep your right foot on the ground and rest your hands on the ground in front of you. Feel the stretch on the inside of your right thigh. Hold the stretch for the prescribed duration and repeat with your left leg.

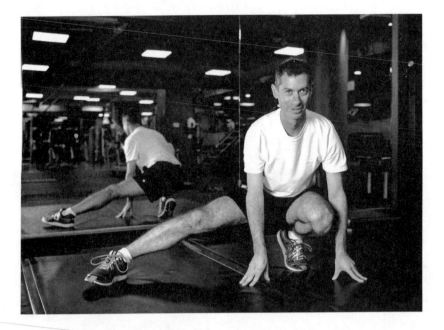

Static Hip Flexor Stretch

Kneel on a soft surface with your right knee on the ground. Bring your left leg in front of you and place your foot flat on the ground so that your knee is positioned over your ankle and bent at 90 degrees. Lean slightly forward until you feel the stretch in your right hip flexor. Hold the stretch for the prescribed duration and repeat with your left leg.

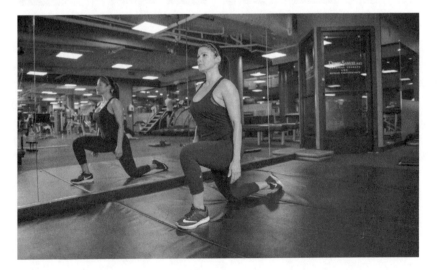

Static Calf Stretch

Stand with your left leg in front of your right leg, hands flat and at shoulder height against a wall. Keep your right leg straight and press your right heel firmly into the ground. Keep your hips facing the wall and your right leg and spine in a straight line. Feel the stretch in the calf of your right leg. Hold the stretch for the prescribed duration and repeat with your left leg.

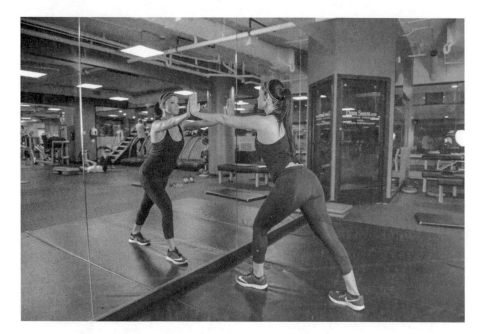

Static Shoulder Stretch

Stand with feet shoulder-width apart. Reach your right arm across your chest, using your left arm to pull your right arm in toward your chest so that you feel the stretch in your right shoulder. Hold the stretch for the prescribed duration and repeat with your left arm.

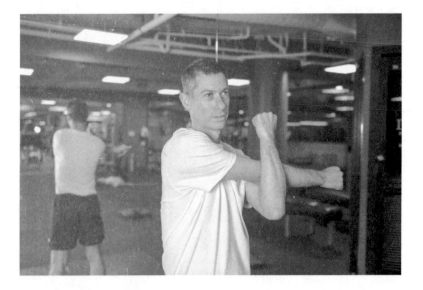

Static Triceps Stretch

Stand with feet shoulder-width apart. Point your right elbow in the air and reach behind you with your right hand to touch your back. With your left hand, reach over your head to grab your right elbow and gently push down on your right elbow to feel the stretch in your right triceps. Hold the stretch for the prescribed duration and repeat with your left arm.

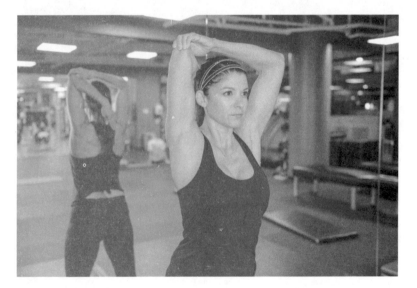

DYNAMIC STRETCHING

Dynamic stretching improves flexibility by using momentum to move your limbs to the edges of their ranges of motion. It also improves body awareness and challenges your balance and coordination.

Dynamic Stretching Workout

Exercise	Reps
Dynamic Glute Stretch	10 each leg
Dynamic Hamstrings Stretch	10 each leg
Dynamic Quadriceps Stretch	10 each leg
Dynamic Adductor Stretch	10 each leg
Dynamic Calf Stretch	10 each leg
Side-to-Side Leg Swings	10 each leg
Forward-and-Back Leg Swings	10 each leg
Lunge and Twist	10 each leg
Arm Circles	10 each arm
Dynamic Shoulder Stretch	10

EXERCISE INSTRUCTIONS

Dynamic Glute Stretch

Lie on your back and bend your right knee, with your left leg straight out in front of you. Place your hands at your sides [1]. Using your abdominals and hip flexors, pull your right leg toward your chest until you can go no farther. Gently assist your leg at the end of the stretch with your hands [2]. Hold the stretch for one to two seconds, return to the starting position, and repeat for the prescribed number of reps before switching to the left leg.

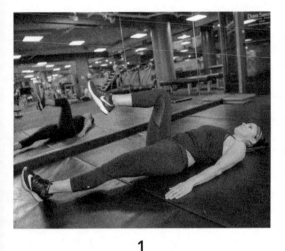

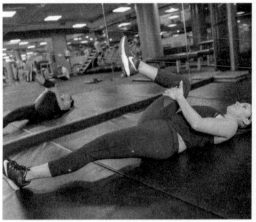

1	**2**

Dynamic Hamstrings Stretch

Lie on your back with your legs straight out in front of you. Make a loop with a rope and place your right foot into the loop [1]. From your hip and using your quadriceps, lift your right leg toward your chest, aiming your foot toward the ceiling. Grasp the ends of the rope with both hands and slightly pull the rope toward you to assist at the end of the stretch [2]. Hold the stretch for one to two seconds, return to the starting position, and repeat for the prescribed number of reps before switching to the left leg.

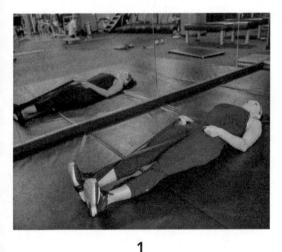

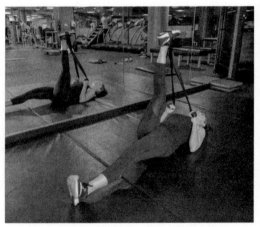

1	**2**

Dynamic Quadriceps Stretch

Lie on your left side in a fetal position with your knees bent. Lay your left arm above your head and your right arm on your right thigh [1]. Reach down with your right hand and grasp your right shin, ankle, or foot and, while contracting your hamstrings and glutes, pull your right leg back as far as you can, using your hand or a rope to give a gentle assistance at the end of the stretch [2]. Hold the stretch for one to two seconds, return to the starting position, and repeat for the prescribed number of reps before switching to the left leg.

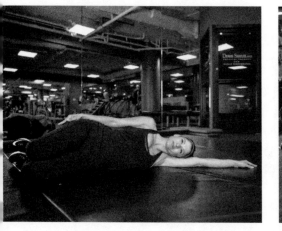

1

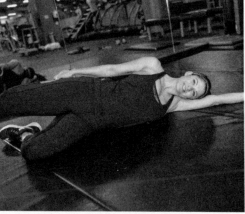

2

Dynamic Adductor Stretch

Lie on your back with both legs extended straight out and loop a rope around the inside of your right ankle and then under your right foot, so the ends of the rope are on the outside of your foot [1]. Extend your right leg out from the side of your body, leading with your heel. Keep slight tension on the rope and use it for gentle assistance at the end of the stretch [2]. Hold the stretch for one to two seconds, return to the starting position, and repeat for the prescribed number of reps before switching to the left leg.

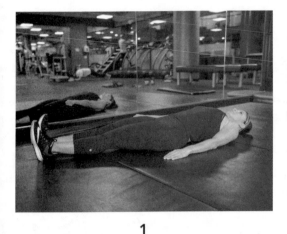

1

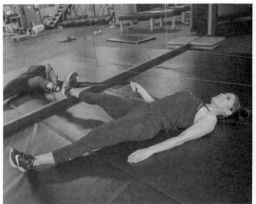

2

Dynamic Calf Stretch

Sit with both legs straight out in front of you and loop a rope around your right foot [1]. Flex your foot back toward you, pulling the rope to assist until you feel slight tension in your calf from the stretch [2]. Hold the stretch for one to two seconds, return to the starting position, and repeat for the prescribed number of reps before switching to the left leg.

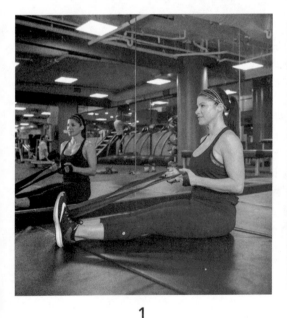

1

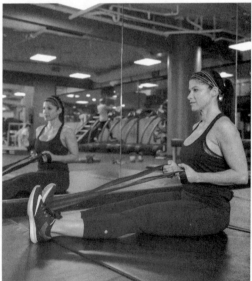

2

Side-to-Side Leg Swings

Stand a couple of feet in front of a wall, chair, or fence with your hands on the wall. Swing your right leg side to side from your hip through its entire range of motion [1], passing your right leg in front of your left leg [2]. Repeat for the prescribed number of reps before switching to the left leg.

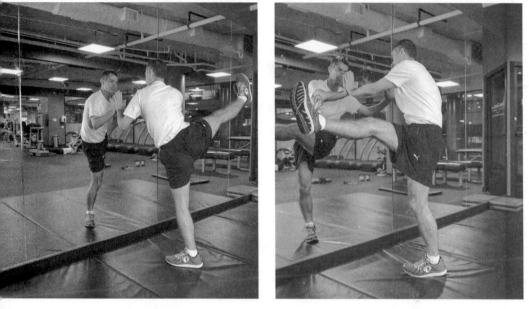

1   2

Forward-and-Back Leg Swings

Stand with the right side of your body facing a wall, chair, or fence with your right hand on the wall. Swing your right leg forward and back from your hip through its entire range of motion [1–2]. Repeat for the prescribed number of reps before switching to the left leg.

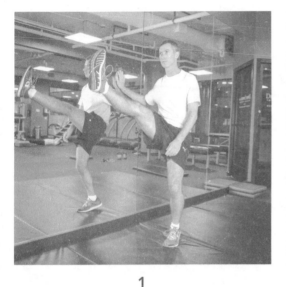

1

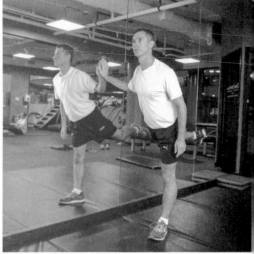

2

Lunge and Twist

Stand with feet shoulder-width apart [1]. Step forward with your right leg like you're doing a lunge, and slowly twist your torso to the right [2]. Then, walk forward, repeating the movement with the left side of your body, lunging with your left leg and slowly twisting your torso to the left. Repeat for the prescribed number of reps with each leg.

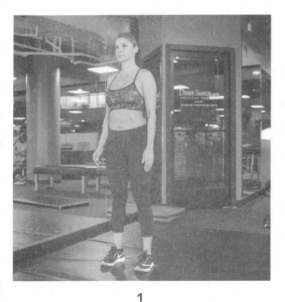

1

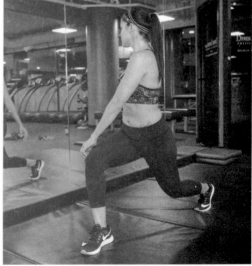

2

Arm Circles

Stand with feet shoulder-width apart, your left arm down to your side, and your right arm straight out to your side with palm facing down [1]. Make circles of about one foot in diameter with your right outstretched arm [2]. Repeat for the prescribed number of reps before switching to the left arm.

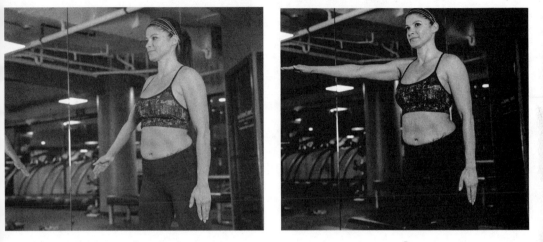

1   2

Dynamic Shoulder Stretch

Stand with feet shoulder-width apart. Grab a towel or Thera-Band at each end and hold it with your arms outstretched in front of you [1]. Keeping your arms straight, raise arms above your head and as far back behind your body as you can go [2]. Repeat for the prescribed number of reps.

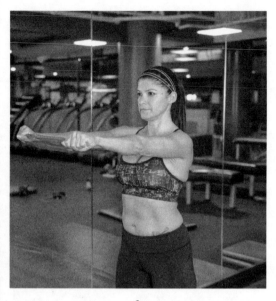
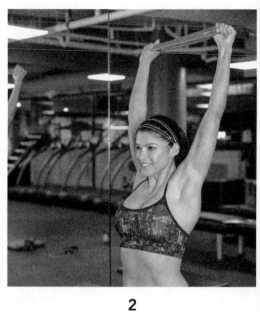

1

2

PROPRIOCEPTIVE NEUROMUSCULAR FACILITATION

A creative method to improve flexibility is a type of stretching given a fancy name—proprioceptive neuromuscular facilitation (PNF), sometimes called precontraction stretching, which exploits a unique property of muscle that causes a muscle to relax after it strongly contracts. Basically, when a lot of tension is developed inside a muscle, a sensory organ that sits at the muscle-tendon junction sends a signal to your central nervous system, which then immediately sends a signal back to the muscle to relax, in order to protect the muscle from damage. With the muscle now relaxed, you can move your limb to a farther point at the end of its range of motion. Thus, your central nervous system facilitates the improvement in flexibility. Pretty cool, huh? For this type of stretching, you'll need a partner to provide resistance as you contract the muscle group being stretched.

PNF Stretching Workout

Exercise	Reps
PNF Hamstrings & Glute Stretch	10 each leg
PNF Quadriceps Stretch	10 each leg
PNF Calf Stretch	10 each leg
PNF Chest/Shoulder Stretch	10

EXERCISE INSTRUCTIONS

PNF Hamstrings & Glute Stretch

Lie with your back on the floor, legs straight, and arms to your sides. Have a partner kneel beside you and lift your right leg up toward your head, keeping your right leg straight so you feel a stretch in your hamstrings. Your partner can rest your leg on his or her shoulder. Keep your left leg flat against the ground [1]. Stretch your hamstrings to the point of limitation, and then contract your hamstrings for a few seconds by pushing your right leg against your partner's resistance, trying to lower your leg [2]. Have your partner restretch your right hamstrings to the point of limitation, which should be slightly farther than the initial stretch [3]. Repeat for the prescribed number of reps before switching to the other leg.

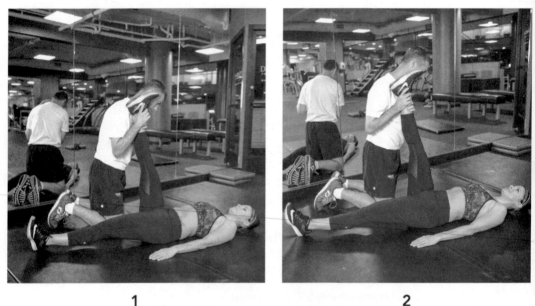

1

2

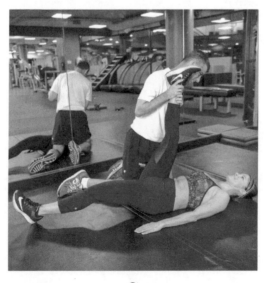

3

PNF Quadriceps Stretch

Lie facedown on the floor with your legs straight and your hands above your head. Have your partner kneel on your right side and bend your right leg until you feel a stretch in your quadriceps. Your partner should have one hand on your quadriceps under your thigh and the other hand on your ankle [1]. Contract your quadriceps for a few seconds by pushing your foot against your partner's resistance, trying to extend your leg [2]. Have your partner restretch your quadriceps to the point of limitation, which should be slightly farther than the initial stretch [3]. Repeat for the prescribed number of reps before switching to the other leg.

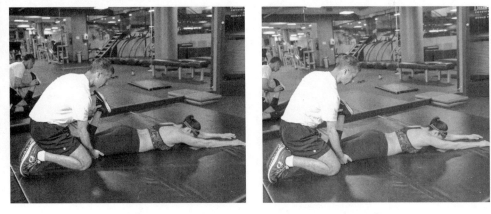

1   2

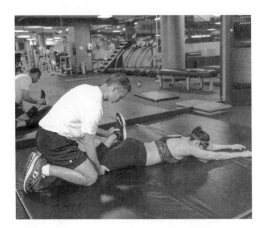

3

PNF Calf Stretch

Sit with your legs out in front of you. Have your partner push the ball of your left foot so that your toes move toward you, stretching your calf [1]. When you reach the point of limitation, contract your calf against your partner's resistance by pushing the ball of your foot against your partner's hand for a few seconds. Relax your calf and allow your partner to push the ball of your foot again to restretch your calf [2]. Repeat for the prescribed number of reps before switching to the other leg.

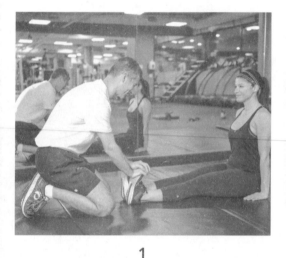
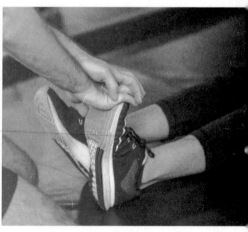

1

2

PNF Chest/Shoulder Stretch

Sit on the ground with legs crossed and arms outstretched to the sides [1]. Your partner stands behind you, grabs your wrists, and gently pulls your arms back to the end of the range of motion [2]. When you reach the point of limitation, contract your chest muscles by trying to pull your arms together against your partner's resistance for a few seconds. Relax your arms and allow your partner to pull them again to restretch your chest and shoulders. Repeat for the prescribed number of reps.

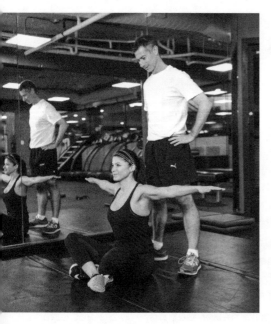
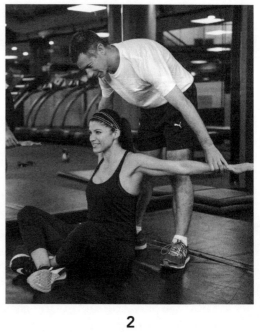

1

2

CHAPTER 6

14-MINUTE METABOLIC WORKOUT MENU

It's one thing to have a collection of awesome workouts in a single book to choose from, but quite another to have a training program that puts them all together so you can become the fittest you've ever been. That's what you get in this chapter. The 14-Minute Metabolic Workout Menu hits all five components of physical fitness with a lot of variety. With a minimum of three workout options for six days per week, the 14-Minute Metabolic Workout Menu gives you at least 729 total weekly combinations so you'll never get bored. Select one option from each day to develop your own unique combination of workouts. If one day you choose an upper-body workout, another day choose a lower-body workout.

The workout menu laid out in this chapter is five courses. Each course has a specific theme and lasts as many weeks as you need to progress at the rate that is right for you, so repeat the week of each course two or three times or as many times as you need until it feels manageable. After you've completed all five courses, return to the first course and slightly increase the intensity of the workouts so you avoid plateaus, continue to adapt, and get fitter.

14-MINUTE METABOLIC WORKOUT MENU

Choose one workout option on each day. All workouts are served with a 5- to 10-minute warm-up and a 5- to 10-minute cool-down. For cardio and sprint workouts, start the warm-up slowly and get progressively faster so you create a smooth transition from warm-up to workout. Finish the warm-up with a few 10-second bursts at the speed/intensity you will use in the workout. For muscular endurance, muscular strength, and muscular power workouts, warm up with a few minutes of cardio and a couple of easy sets of the specific exercises.

Course 1: Muscular Endurance

Monday
Machine Workout

Upper Body 1: Back & Biceps

Upper Body 2: Chest, Shoulders, & Triceps

Lower Body 1: Quads & Calves

Lower Body 2: Hamstrings, Glutes, & Inner Thighs

Total Body Machine Workout

Tuesday

Static Stretching Workout

Dynamic Stretching Workout

PNF Stretching Workout

Wednesday
Circuit Workout

Dumbbell Total-Body Circuit

Sprint/Body Weight Circuit

Core Circuit

Resistance Band Circuit

Kettlebell Circuit

TRX Circuit

Short Circuit 1

Short Circuit 2

Short Circuit 3

Thursday

Rest Day

Friday

Dumbbell Workout

Upper Body 1: Back & Biceps

Upper Body 2: Chest, Shoulders, & Triceps

Lower Body 1: Quads & Calves

Lower Body 2: Hamstrings, Glutes, & Inner Thighs

Total Body Dumbbell Workout

Saturday

Static Stretching Workout

Dynamic Stretching Workout

PNF Stretching Workout

Sunday

Body Weight Workout

Upper Body 1: Back & Abs

Upper Body 2: Chest, Shoulders, & Triceps

Lower Body 1: Quads & Calves

Lower Body 2: Hamstrings, Glutes, & Inner Thighs

Total Body Weight Workout

Monday

VO$_2$max Workout

VO$_2$max 5 x 1

VO$_2$max 4 x 2

VO$_2$max 3 x 3

VO$_2$max 2 x 5

VO$_2$max Alternating 1–2

VO$_2$max Ladder

VO$_2$max Pyramid

Tuesday

Static Stretching Workout

Dynamic Stretching Workout

PNF Stretching Workout

Wednesday

Aerobic Tempo Workout

Aerobic Tempo 5 x 2

Aerobic Tempo 3 x 4

Aerobic Tempo 2 x 6

Continuous Aerobic Tempo

Thursday

Rest Day

Friday

Treadmill Hill Workout

Treadmill Hill Pyramid 1

Treadmill Hill Pyramid 2

Treadmill Hill Ladder

Treadmill Triple 3 Hills

Saturday

Static Stretching Workout

Dynamic Stretching Workout

PNF Stretching Workout

Sunday

Fartlek Workout

Classic Fartlek

1–2–3–2–1 Fartlek

3–2–2–3 Fartlek

4–3–2–1-½ Fartlek

Course 3: Muscular Strength

Monday

Hypertrophy Machine Workout

Upper Body 1: Back & Biceps

Upper Body 2: Chest, Shoulders, & Triceps

Lower Body 1: Quads & Calves

Lower Body 2: Hamstrings & Glutes

Upper Body Strength Pyramid

Lower Body Strength Pyramid

Upper Body Drop Sets

Lower Body Drop Sets

Total Body Machine Workout

Tuesday

Static Stretching Workout

Dynamic Stretching Workout

PNF Stretching Workout

Wednesday

Neuromuscular Machine Workout

Upper Body 1: Chest & Triceps

Upper Body 2: Back & Biceps

Lower Body 1: Quads & Calves

Lower Body 2: Hamstrings & Glutes

Total Body Machine Workout

Thursday

Rest Day

Friday

Hypertrophy Dumbbell Workout

Upper Body 1: Back & Biceps

Upper Body 2: Chest, Shoulders, & Triceps

Lower Body 1: Quads & Calves

Lower Body 2: Hamstrings, Glutes, & Inner Thighs

Total Body Dumbbell Workout

Saturday

Static Stretching Workout

Dynamic Stretching Workout

PNF Stretching Workout

Sunday

Neuromuscular Dumbbell Workout

Upper Body 1: Chest & Triceps

Upper Body 2: Back & Biceps

Lower Body 1: Quads & Calves

Lower Body 2: Hamstrings & Glutes

Total Body Dumbbell Workout

Course 4: Sprint

Monday

Sprint Workout

Sprint 10 x 10

Sprint 10 x 20

Sprint 10 x 30

Tuesday

Static Stretching Workout

Dynamic Stretching Workout

PNF Stretching Workout

Wednesday

Sprint Workout

Sprint 5 x 1

Sprint Ladder

Sprint Pyramid

True Tabata

Thursday

Rest Day

Friday

Sprint Workout

Sprint 10 x 10

Sprint 10 x 20

Sprint 10 x 30

Saturday

Static Stretching Workout

Dynamic Stretching Workout

PNF Stretching Workout

Sunday

Sprint Workout

Sprint 5 x 1

Sprint Ladder

Sprint Pyramid

True Tabata

Course 5: Muscular Power

Monday

Machine Workout

Upper Body 1: Back & Biceps

Upper Body 2: Chest, Shoulders, & Triceps

Lower Body 1: Quads & Calves

Lower Body 2: Hamstrings, Glutes, & Inner Thighs

Total Body Machine Workout

Tuesday

Static Stretching Workout

Dynamic Stretching Workout

PNF Stretching Workout

Wednesday

Plyometric Workout

Plyometric Power Workout

Power Circuit

Thursday

Rest Day

Friday

Machine Workout

Upper Body 1: Back & Biceps

Upper Body 2: Chest, Shoulders, & Triceps

Lower Body 1: Quads & Calves

Lower Body 2: Hamstrings, Glutes, & Inner Thighs

Total Body Machine Workout

Saturday

Static Stretching Workout

Dynamic Stretching Workout

PNF Stretching Workout

Sunday

Plyometric Workout

Plyometric Power Workout

Power Circuit

ABOUT THE AUTHOR

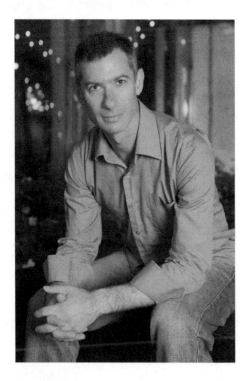

A runner since age eleven, Dr. Jason Karp is one of America's foremost running experts, an entrepreneur, and the creator of the Revo$_2$lution Running™ certification. He owns Run-Fit, LLC, the premier provider of innovative running and fitness services. He has been profiled in a number of publications and is the 2011 IDEA Personal Trainer of the Year (the fitness industry's highest award) and 2014 recipient of the President's Council on Fitness, Sports & Nutrition Community Leadership Award.

Dr. Karp has given hundreds of national and international lectures and has been a featured speaker at the world's top fitness conferences and coaching clinics, including Asia Fitness Convention, Indonesia Fitness & Health Expo, FILEX Fitness Convention (Australia), U.S. Track & Field and Cross Country Coaches Association Convention, American College of Sports

Medicine Conference, IDEA World Fitness Convention, SCW Fitness MANIA, National Strength & Conditioning Association Conference, ECA World Fitness Convention, and CanFitPro, among others. He has been an instructor for USA Track & Field's level 3 coaching certification and for coaching camps at the U.S. Olympic Training Center.

A prolific writer, Jason is the author of seven other books: *Run Your Fat Off, The Inner Runner, Running a Marathon For Dummies, Running for Women, 101 Winning Racing Strategies for Runners, 101 Developmental Concepts & Workouts for Cross Country Runners*, and *How to Survive Your PhD*, and he is the editor of the sixth edition of *Track & Field Omnibook*. He also has more than 400 articles published in a wide variety of international coaching, running, and fitness magazines, including *Track Coach, Techniques for Track & Field and Cross Country, New Studies in Athletics, Runner's World, Running Times, Women's Running, Marathon & Beyond, IDEA Fitness Journal, Oxygen, SELF, Shape*, and *Active.com*, among others.

At age twenty-four, Dr. Karp became one of the youngest college head coaches in the country, leading the Georgian Court University women's cross country team to the regional championship and winning honors as NAIA Northeast Region Coach of the Year. He has also coached high school track and field and cross country. His personal training experience ranges from elite athletes to cardiac rehab patients. As a coach, he has helped many runners meet their potential, ranging from a first-time race participant to an Olympic Trials qualifier. A competitive runner since sixth grade, Dr. Karp is a nationally certified running coach through USA Track & Field, has been sponsored by PowerBar and Brooks, and was a member of the silver medal–winning United States masters half-marathon team at the 2013 World Maccabiah Games in Israel.

Dr. Karp received his PhD in exercise physiology with a physiology minor from Indiana University in 2007, his master's degree in kinesiology from the University of Calgary in 1997, and his bachelor's degree in exercise and sport science with an English minor from Penn State University in 1995. His research has been published in the scientific journals *Medicine & Science in Sports & Exercise, International Journal of Sport Nutrition and Exercise Metabolism,* and *International Journal of Sports Physiology and Performance.*